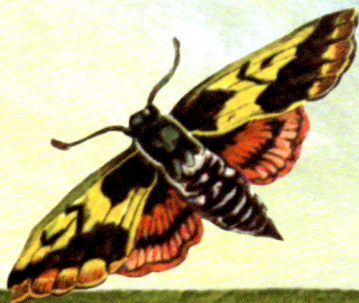

has

anyone

seen

my

hormones?

has anyone seen my hormones?

and other hot flashes of wisdom

from menopause and midlife

by anne taintor

CHRONICLE BOOKS
SAN FRANCISCO

Library of Congress Cataloging-in-Publication Data available.

ISBN 978-1-7972-4109-8

Manufactured in China.

FSC
www.fsc.org

MIX
Paper | Supporting
responsible forestry
FSC™ C008047

Design by Barbara Bersche.

10 9 8 7 6 5 4 3 2 1

Chronicle books and gifts are available at special quantity
discounts to corporations, professional associations, literacy
programs, and other organizations. For details and discount
information, please contact our premiums department at
corporategifts@chroniclebooks.com or at 1-800-759-0190.

Chronicle Books LLC
680 Second Street
San Francisco, California 94107
www.chroniclebooks.com

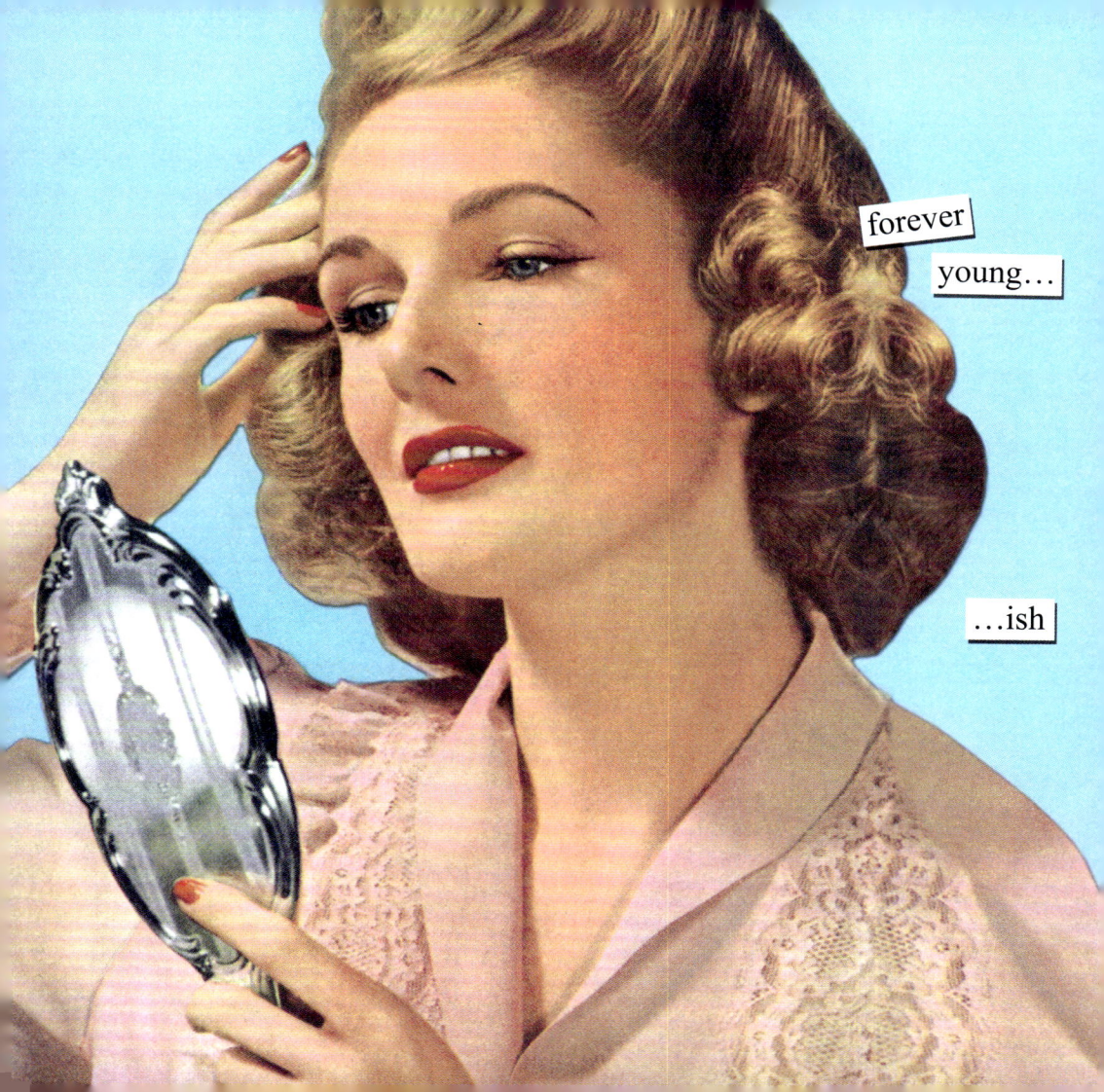

forever

young…

…ish

introduction

Youth wasn't awful.

I vaguely remember having a wrinkle-free neck.

That was nice.

But maturity kicks youth's *ass*!

Aging is an upgrade, not a downgrade.

It's our permission slip to roll our eyes at all the noise and nonsense of our younger years.

It's our time to live boldly, to stop apologizing, and to laugh more loudly.

It's our license to stop giving a rat's ass.

I won't claim that—wise as I may now have become—I don't still occasionally feel a glimmer of insecurity.

I do.

I have not yet attained perfection.

But I've come to the realization that perfection is way, way, *way* overrated.

A wise man once said, "I yam what I yam."

And I'm down with that.

There comes a time in every woman's life when she realizes, "honey, you couldn't *pay* me to be twenty!"

Whether you're still technically young, or whether you're radiantly young-ish . . .

whether you know precisely where your hormones are, or whether you could use a bit of help locating them . . .

whether you're still slogging through the labyrinth we call youth, or whether you have emerged victorious at the glorious, liberating reality of midlife . . .

this book celebrates you!

My friends, you kick ass!

—Anne Taintor

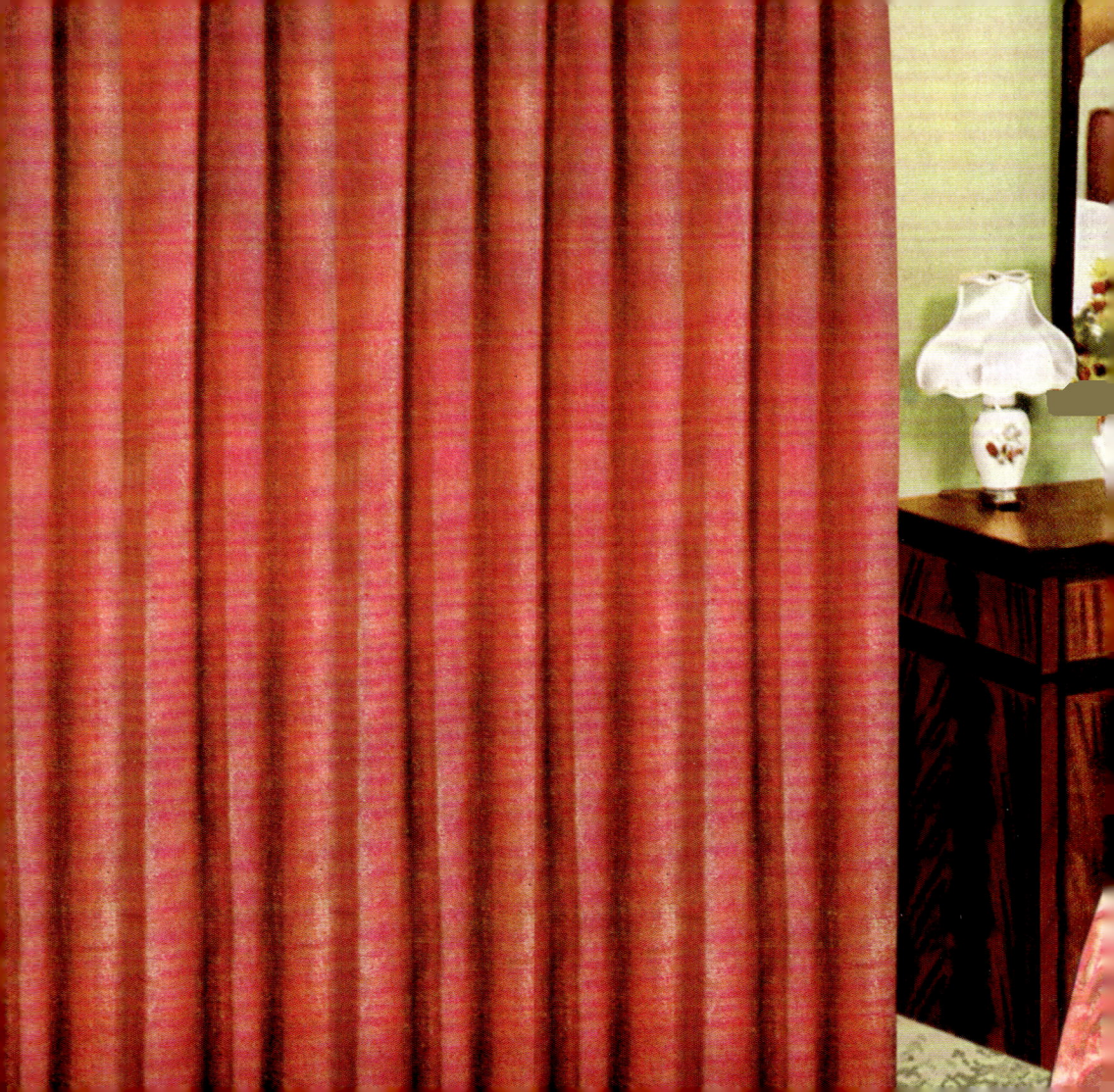

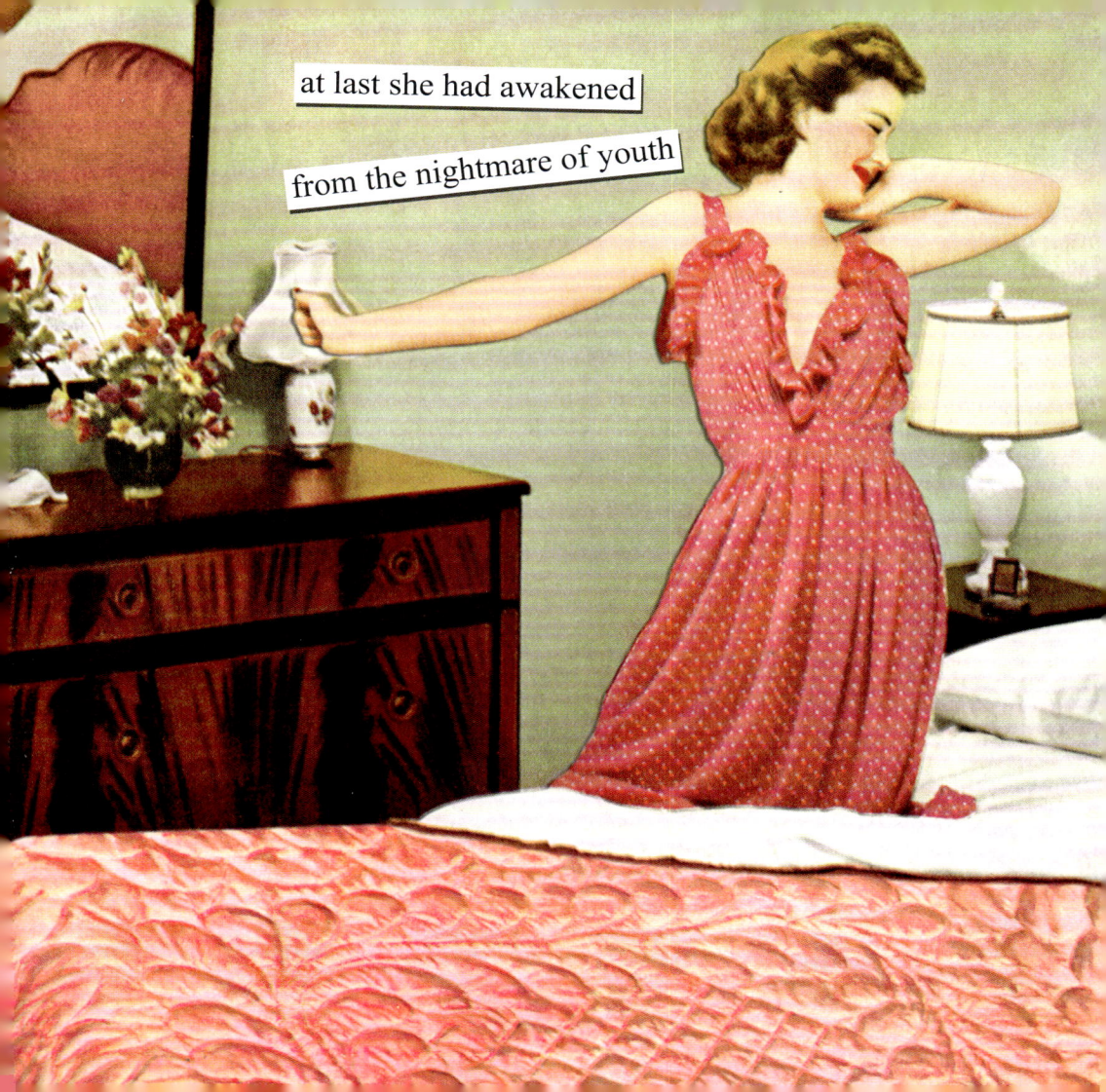

at last she had awakened

from the nightmare of youth

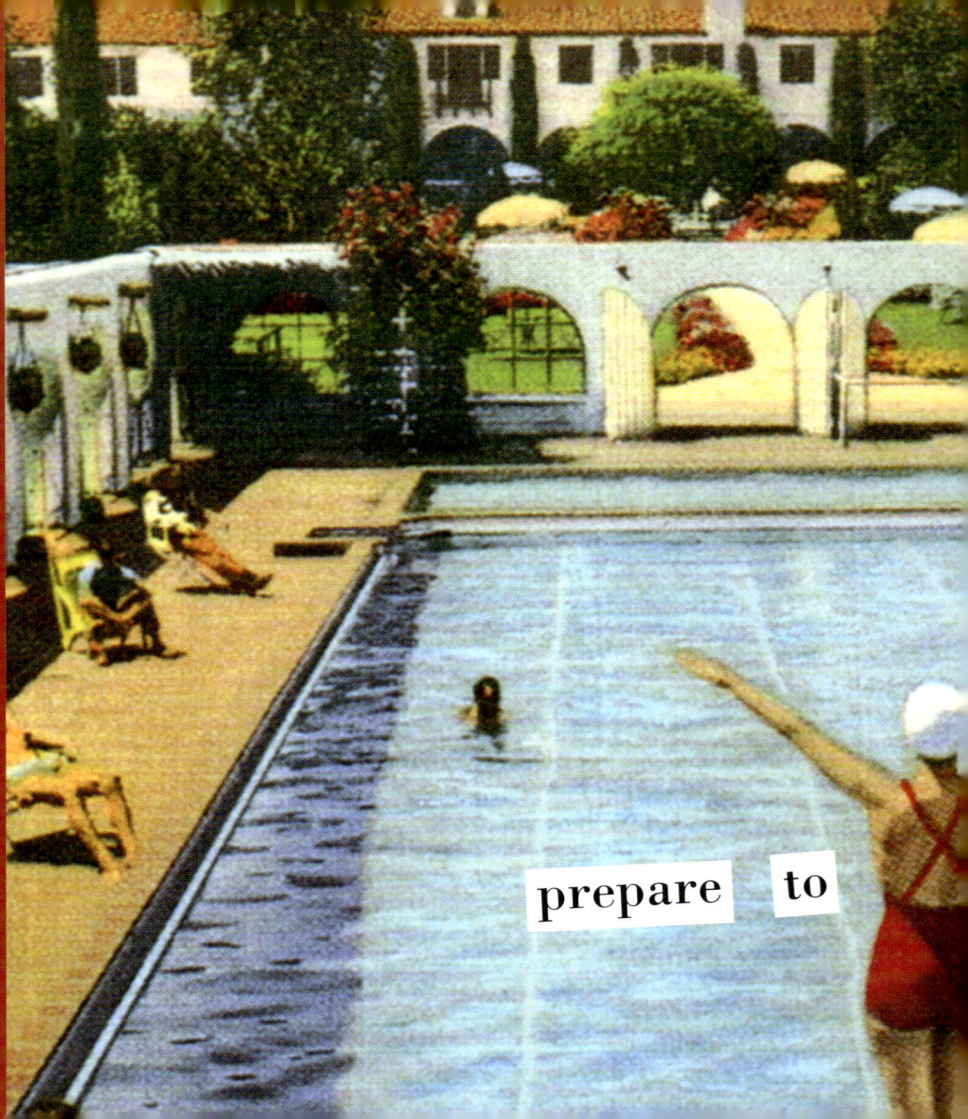

prepare to

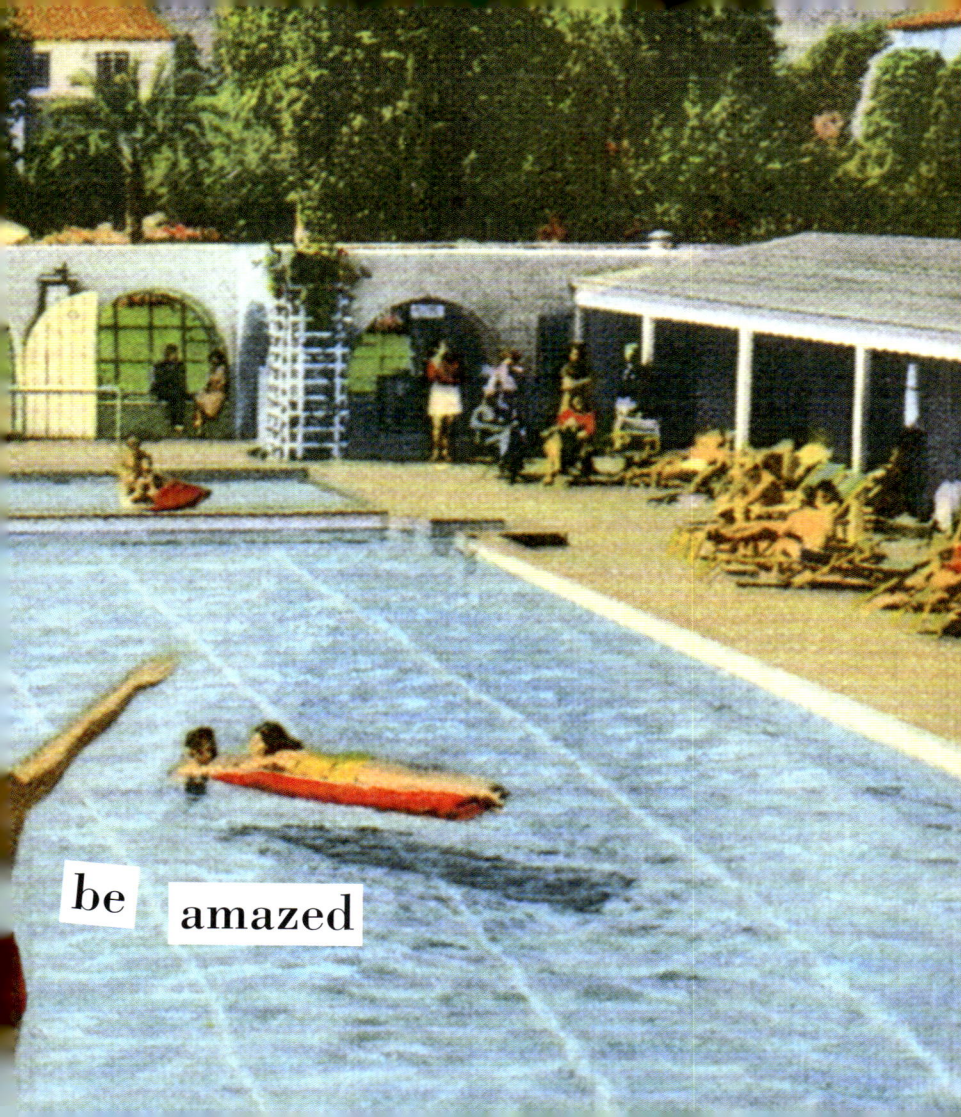

be amazed

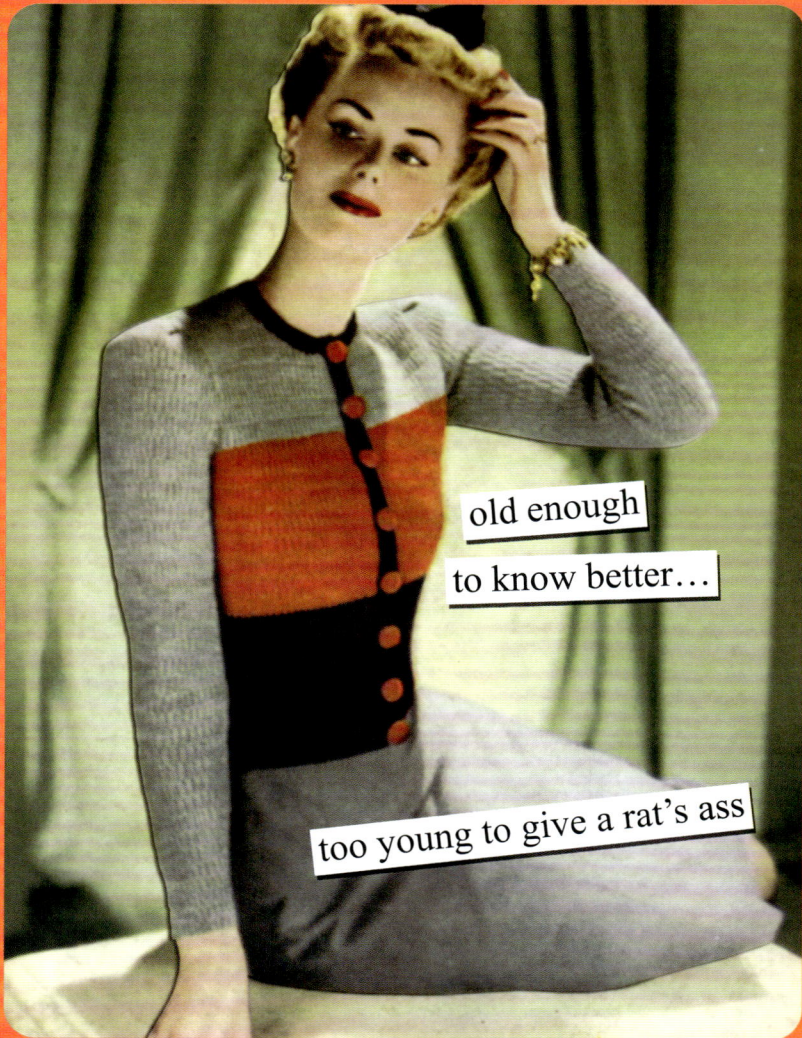

old enough

to know better...

too young to give a rat's ass

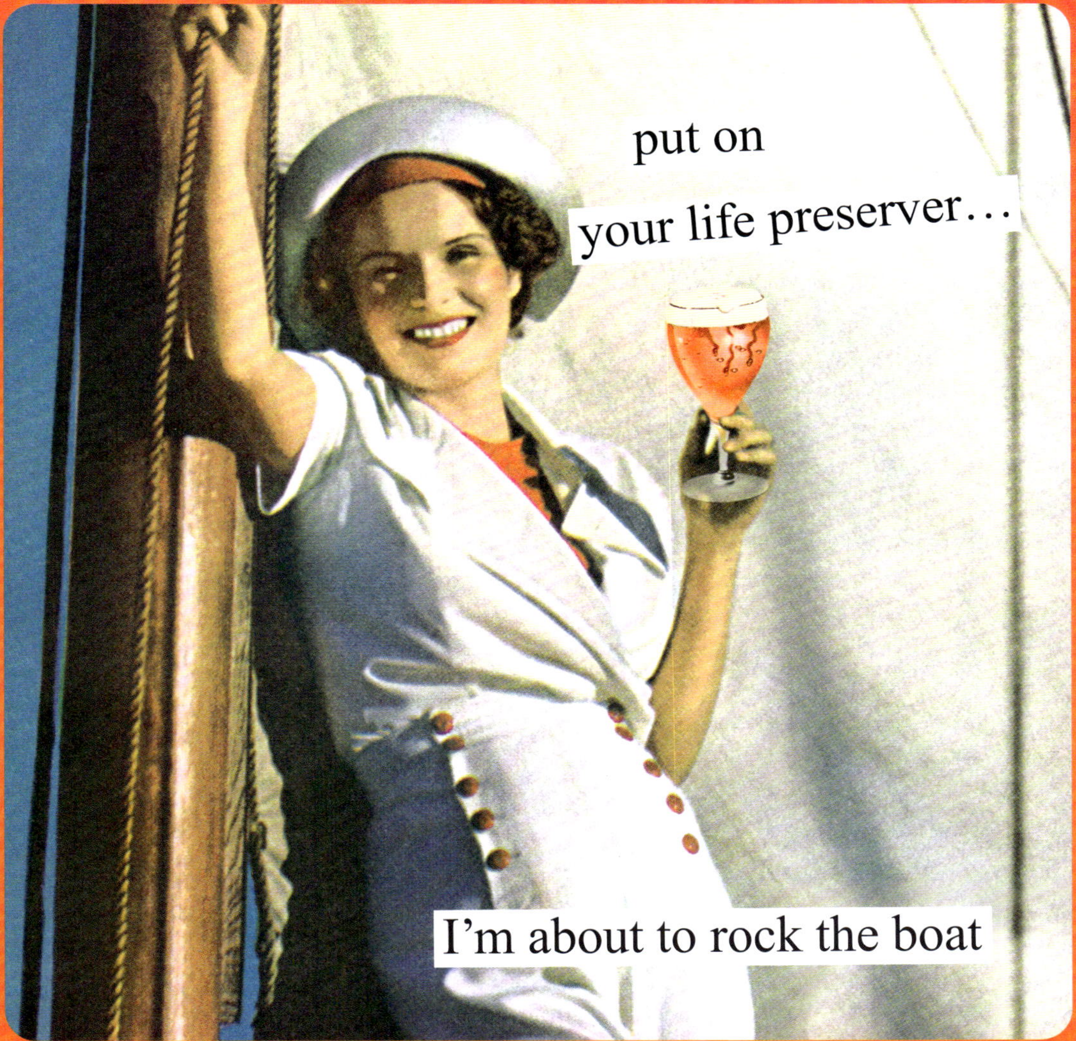
put on
your life preserver…
I'm about to rock the boat

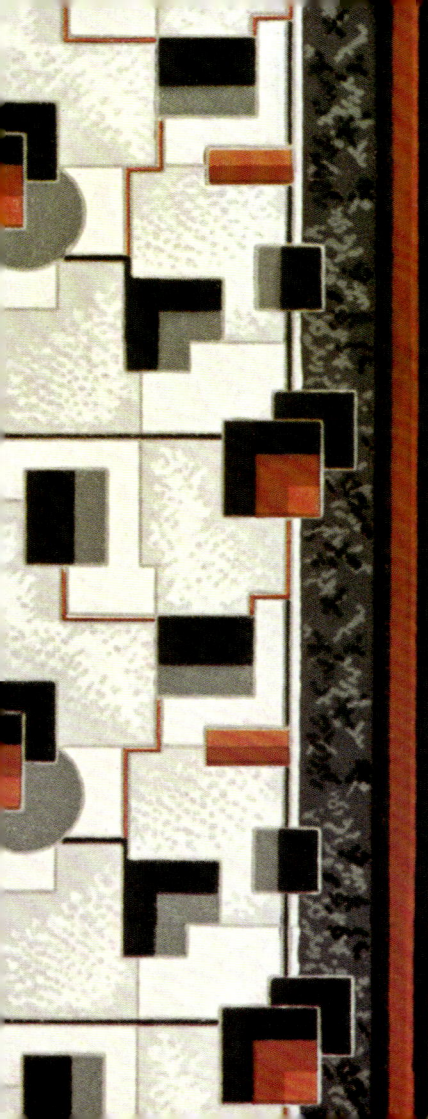

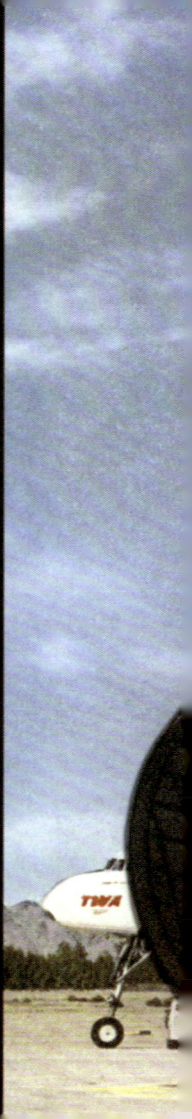

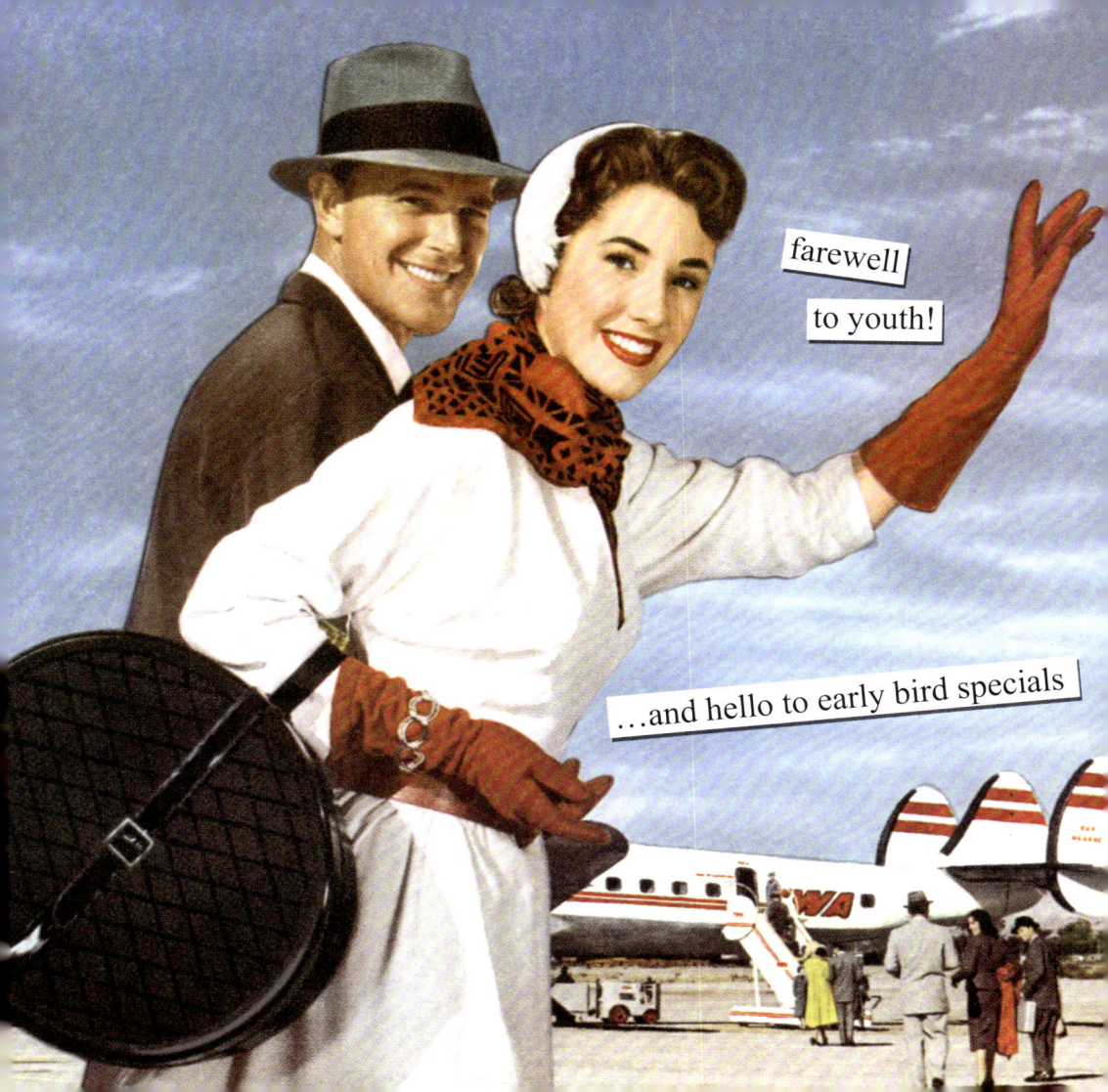

farewell
to youth!

...and hello to early bird specials

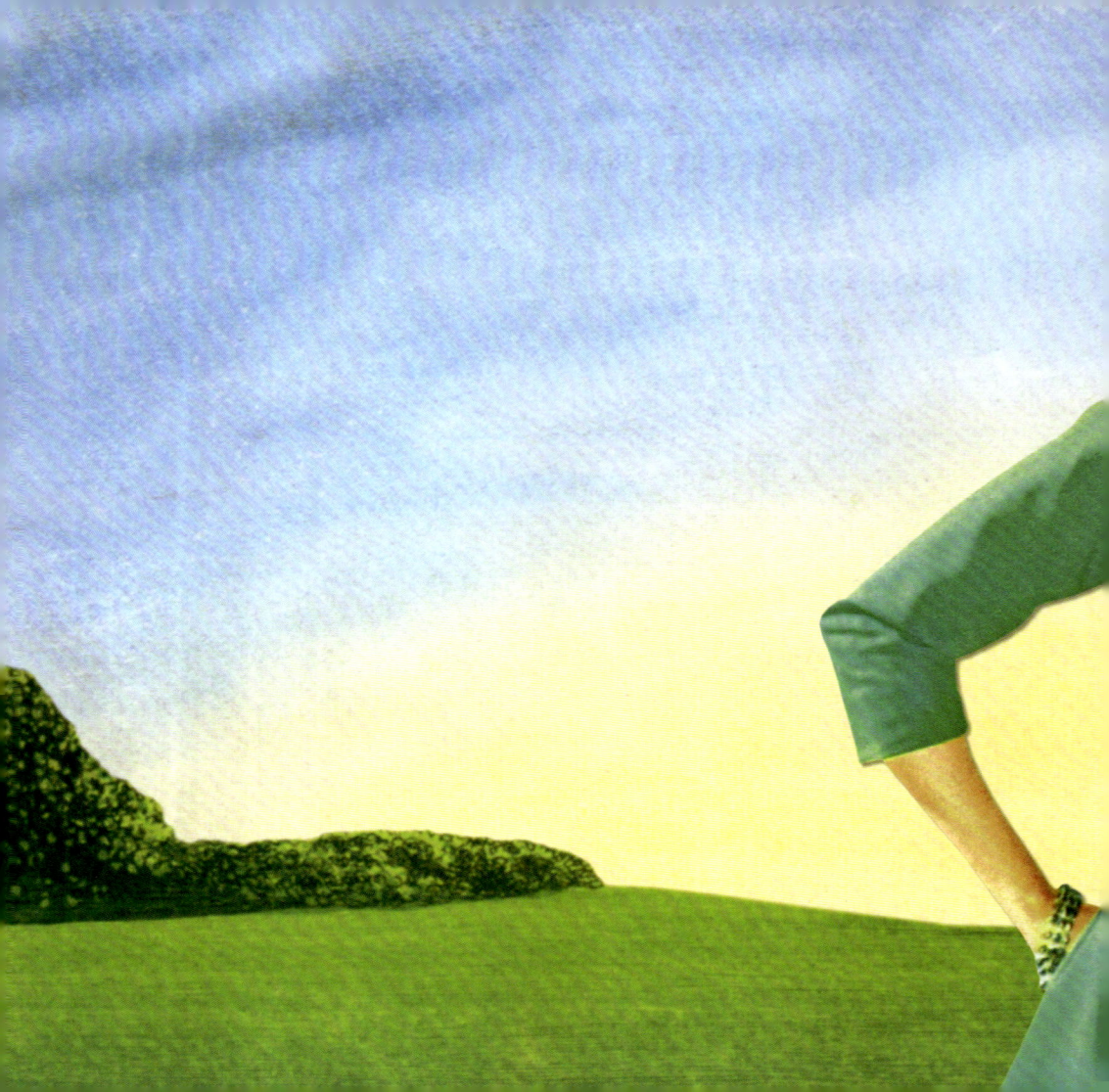

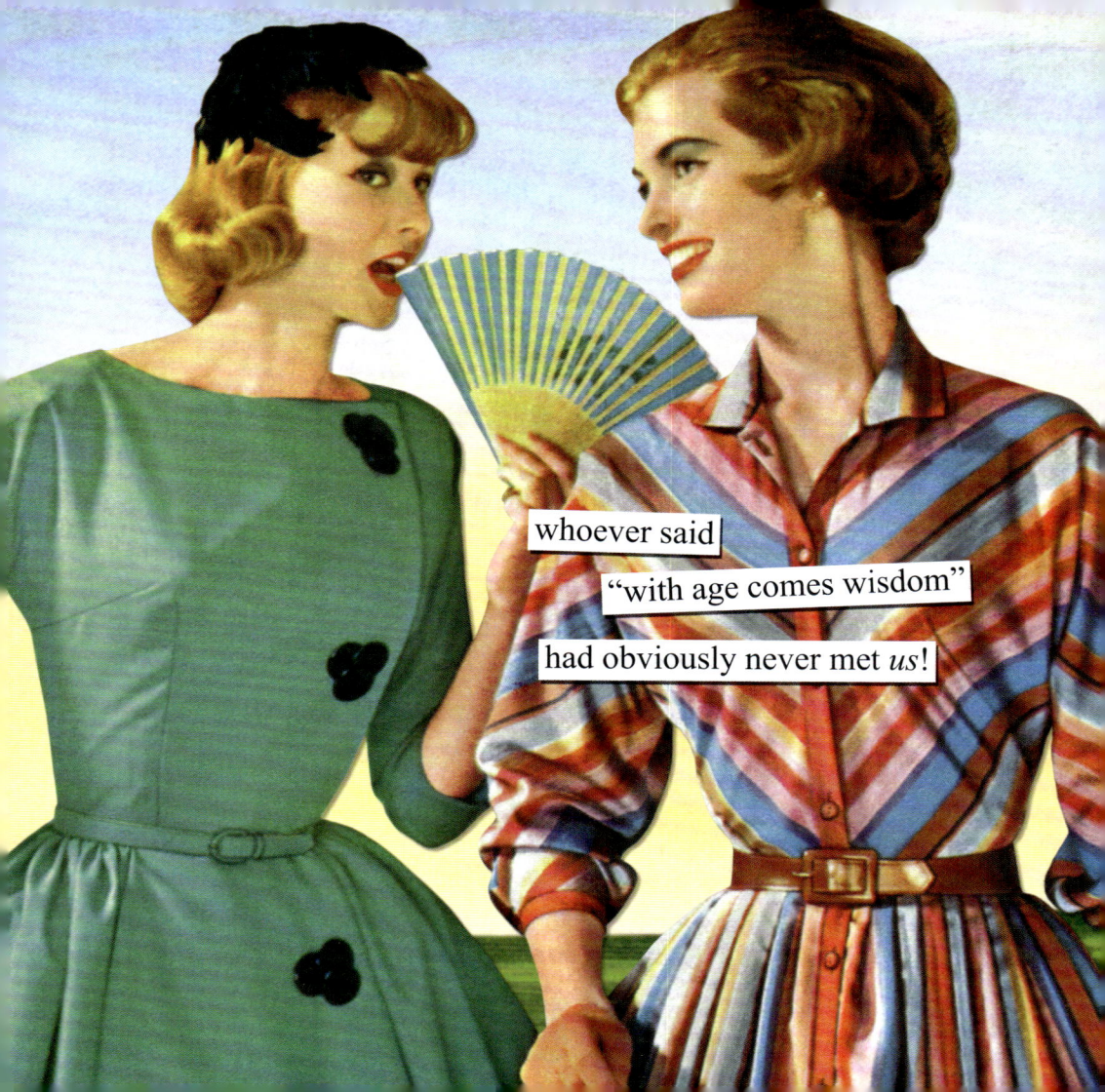

whoever said
"with age comes wisdom"
had obviously never met *us*!

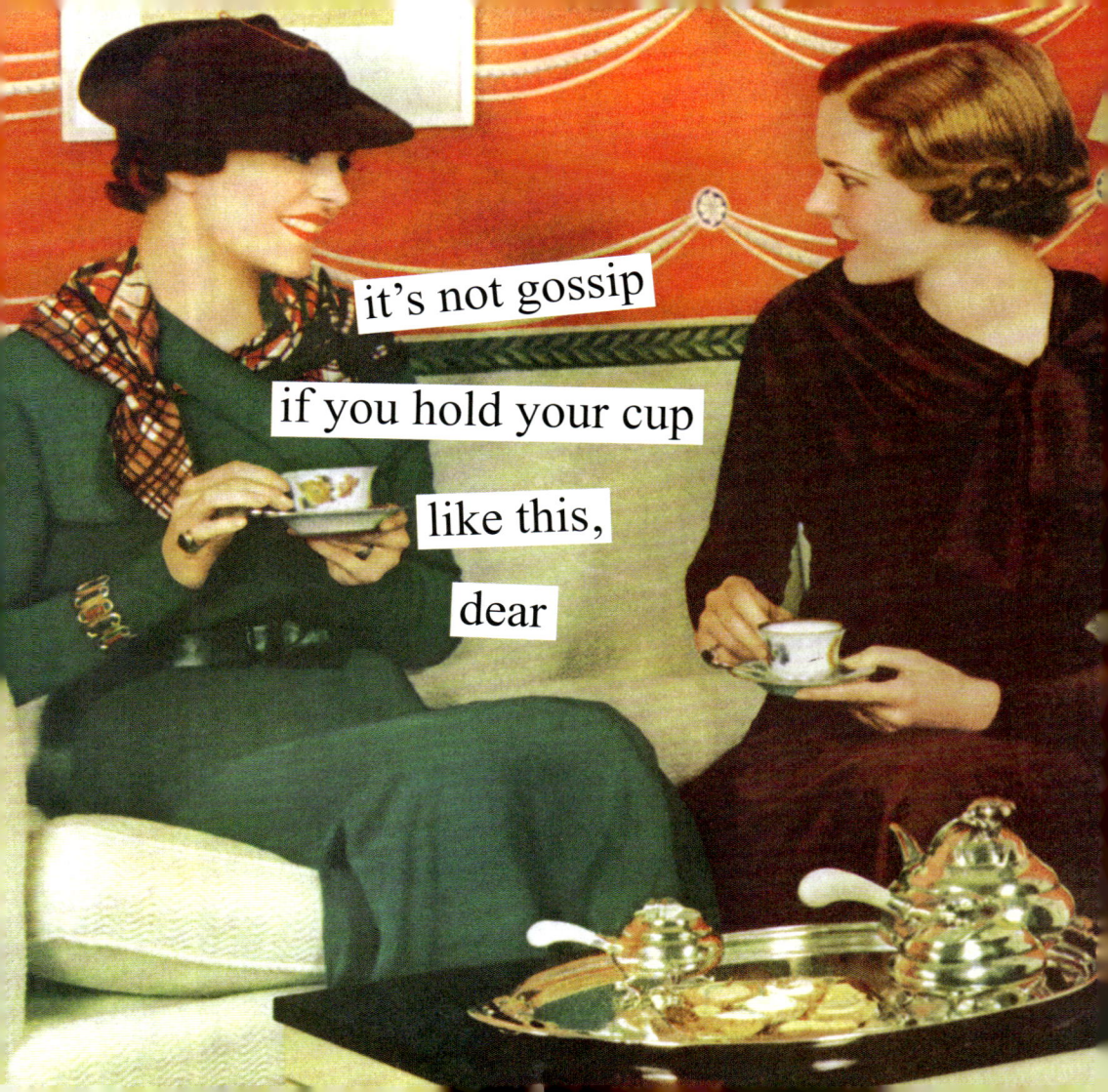

it's not gossip

if you hold your cup

like this,

dear

we prefer "coven"

but "book club" is fine too

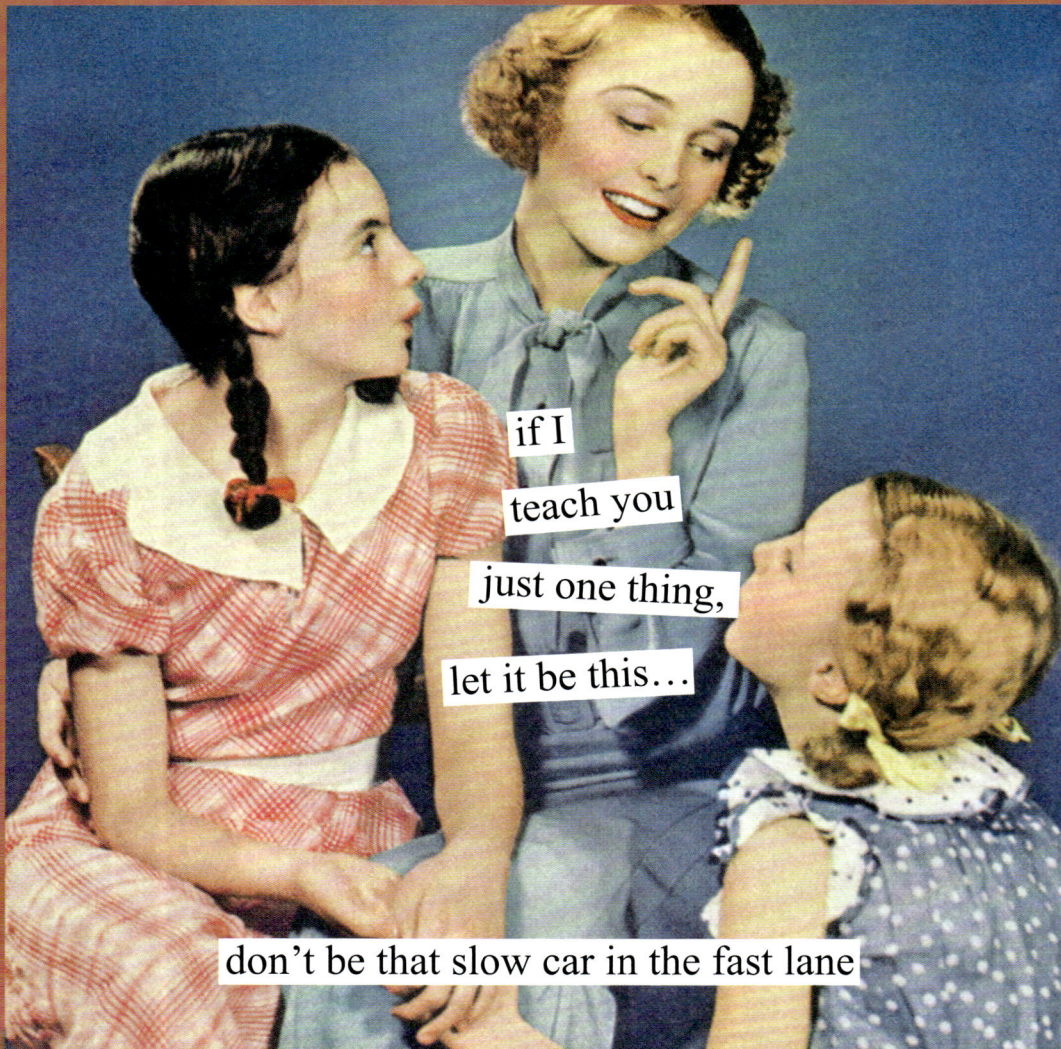

if you're going to kick ass,

you need kickass shoes

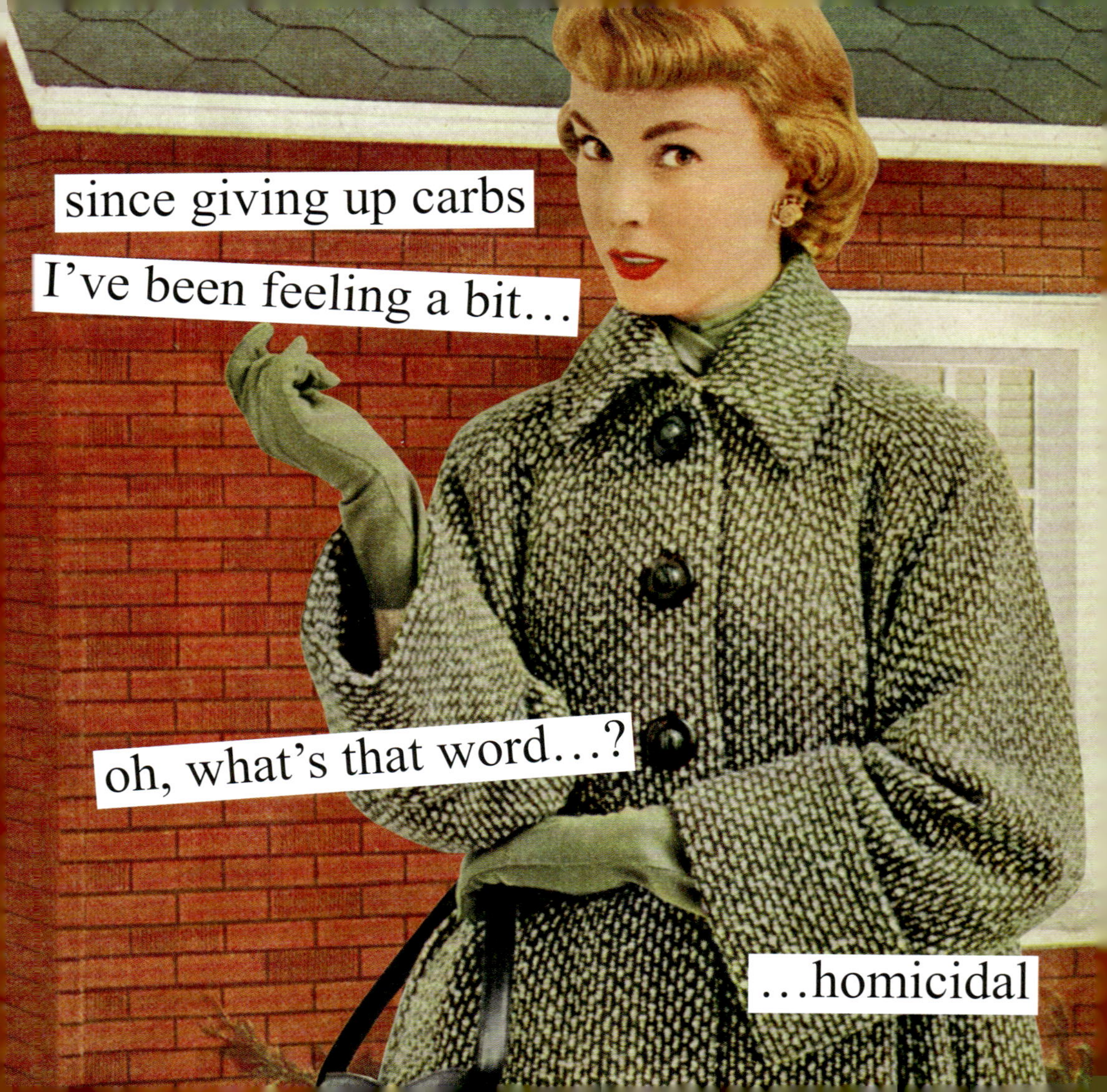
since giving up carbs
I’ve been feeling a bit…
oh, what’s that word…?
…homicidal

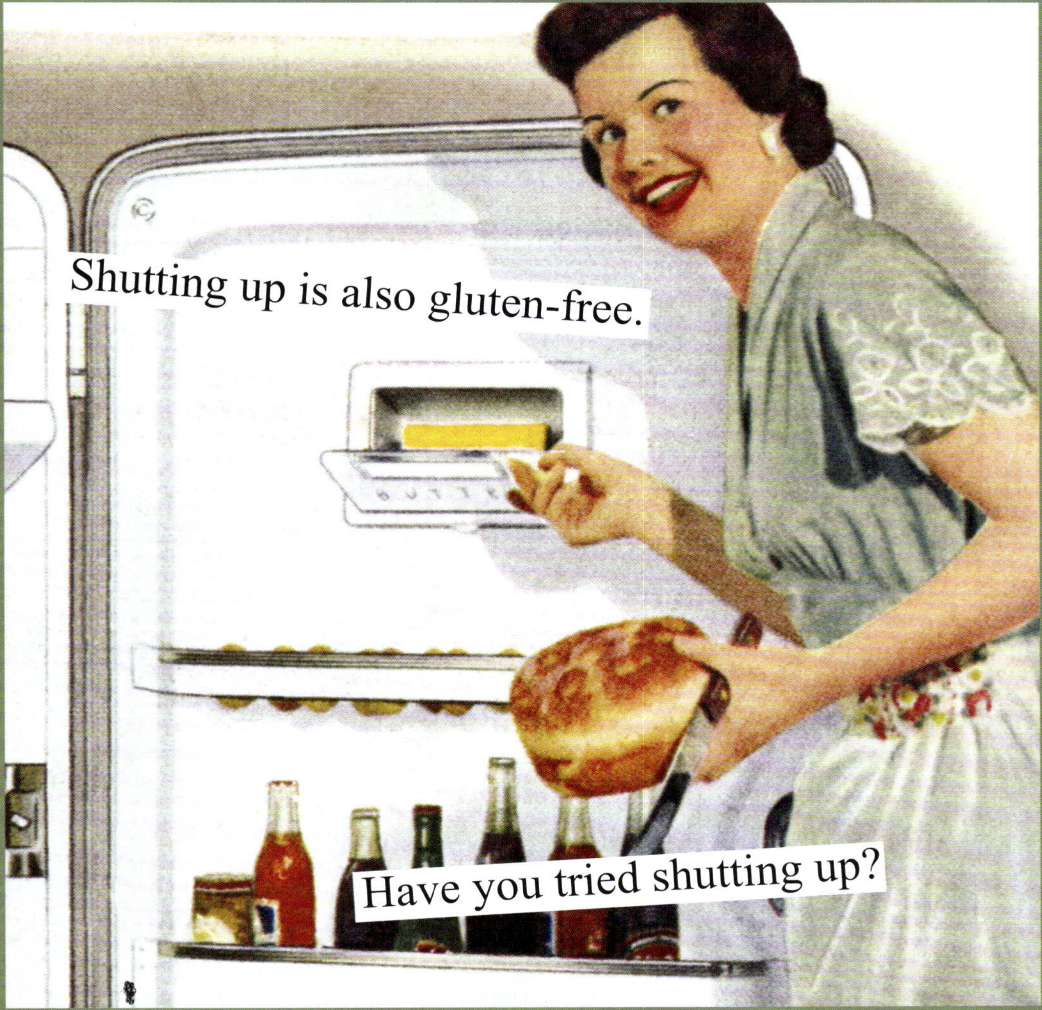
Shutting up is also gluten-free.
Have you tried shutting up?

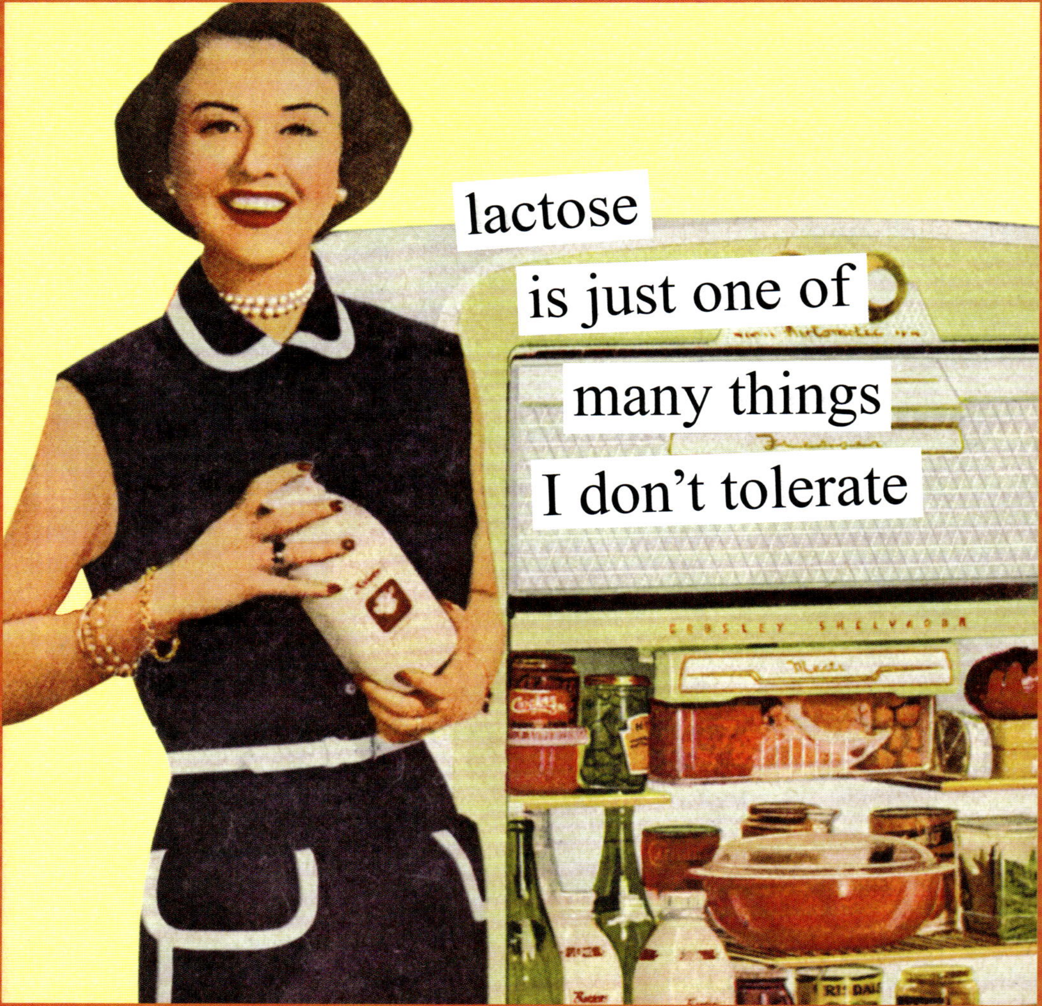

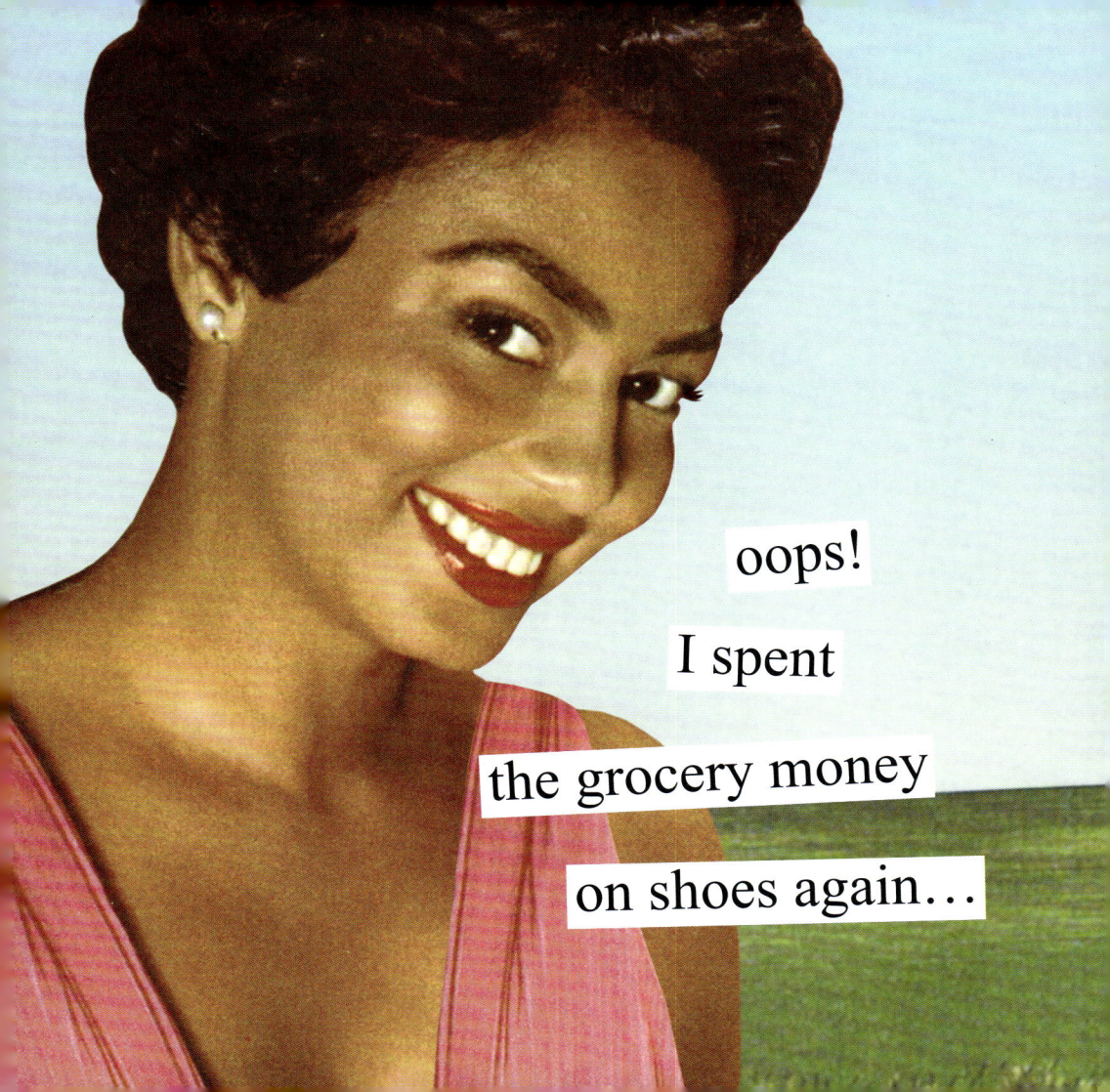

oops!

I spent

the grocery money

on shoes again…

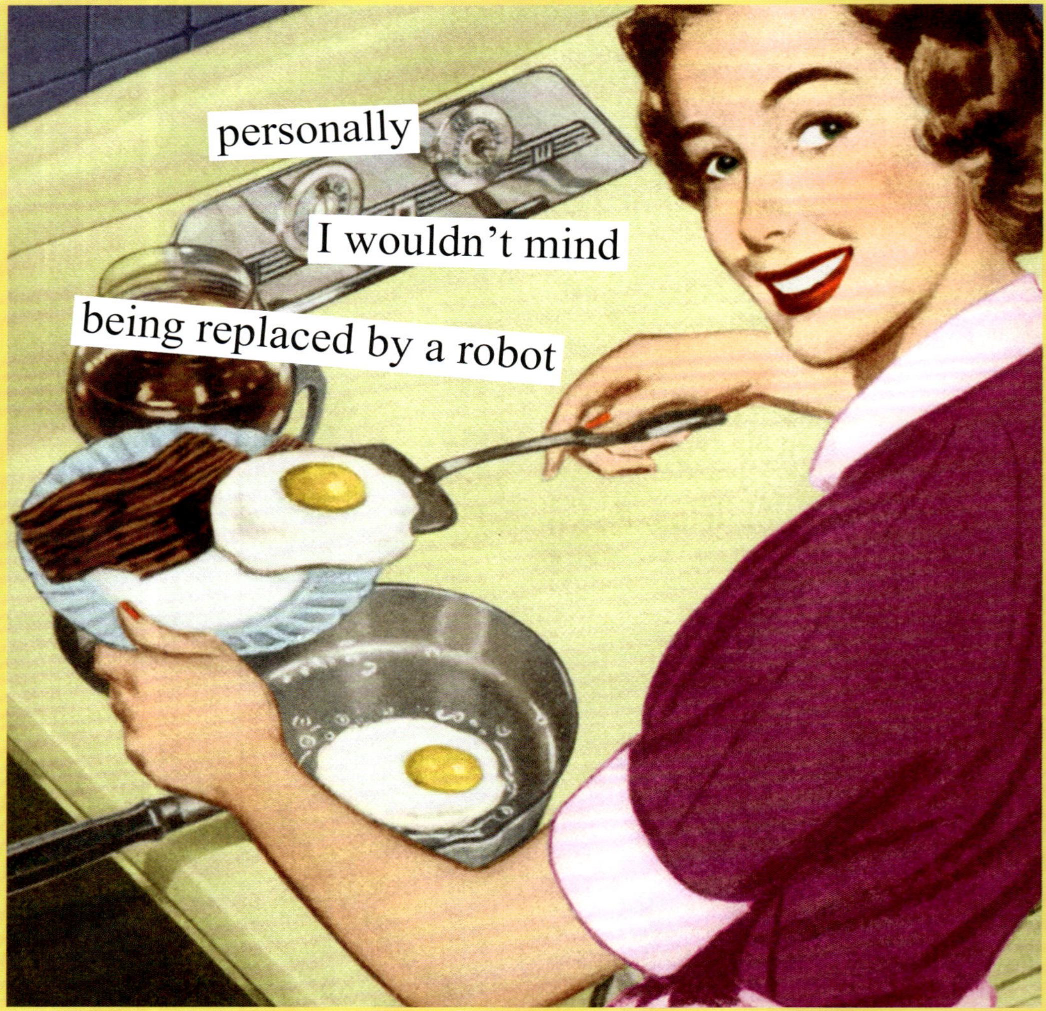
personally
I wouldn't mind
being replaced by a robot

you say

"lazy"

like

it's

a *bad* thing

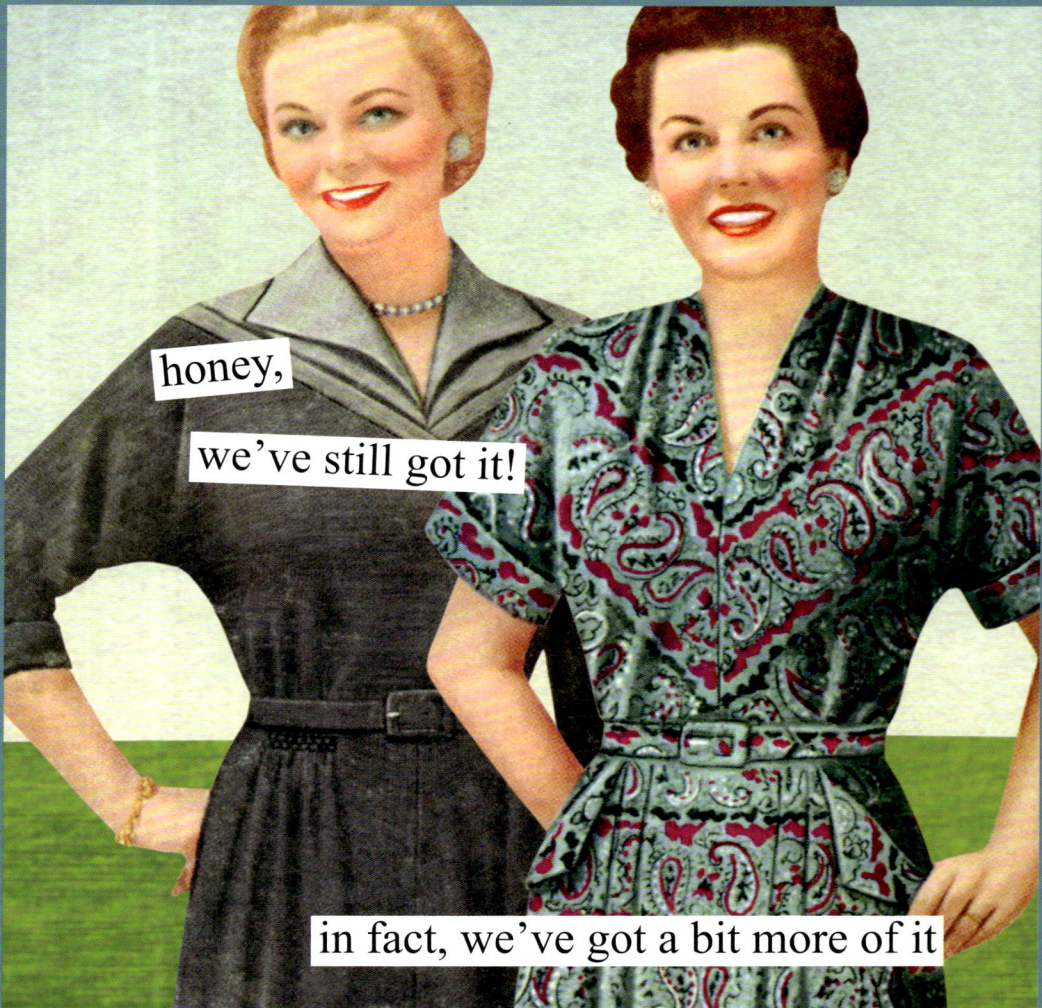

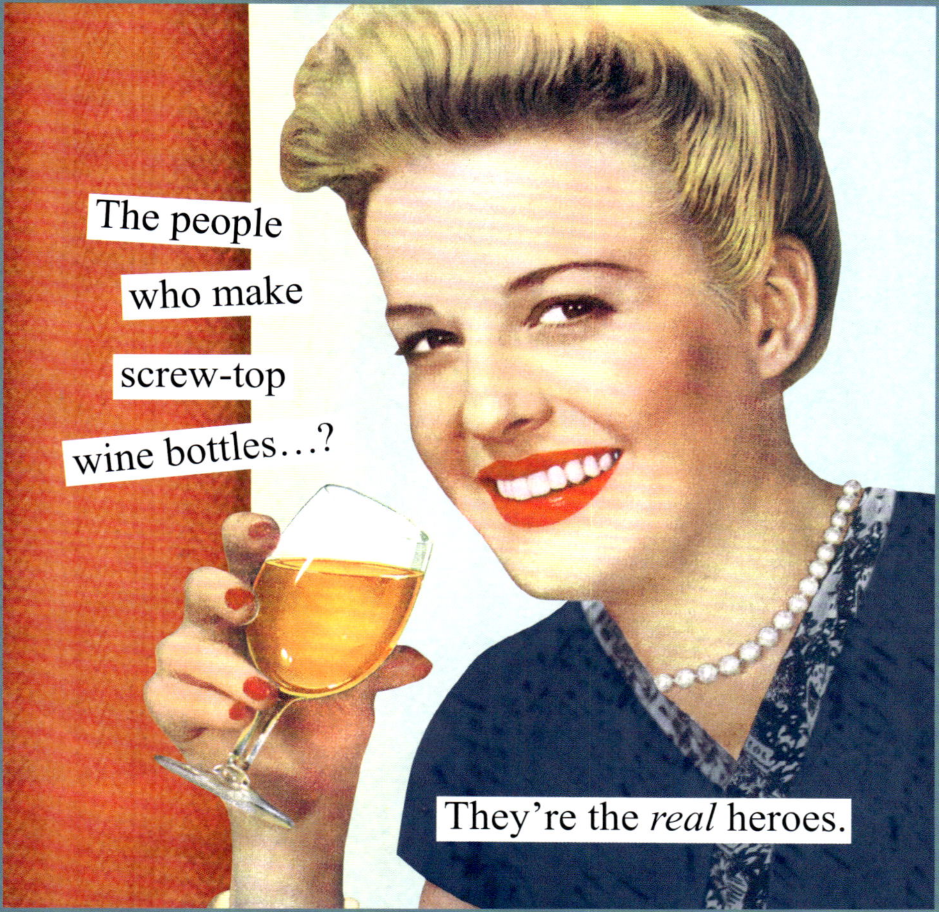
The people
who make
screw-top
wine bottles…?
They’re the *real* heroes.

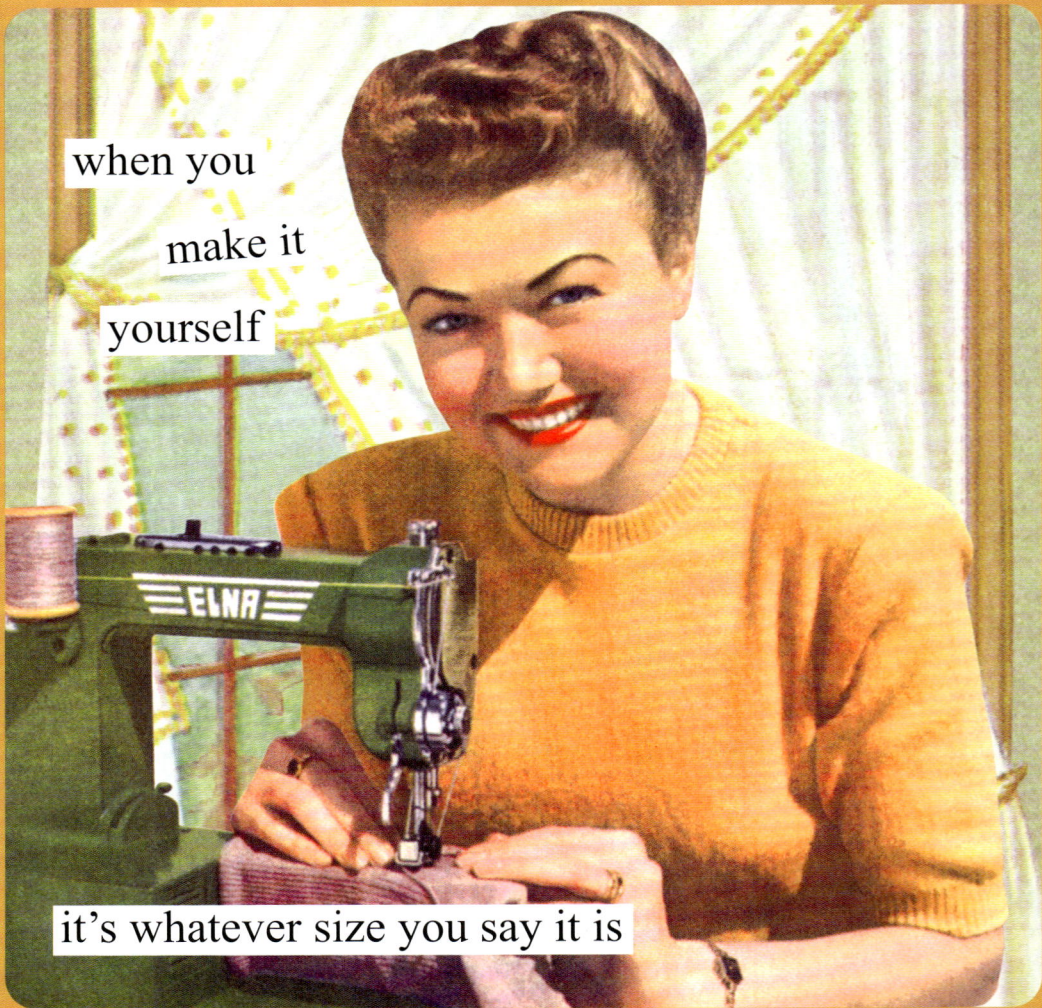

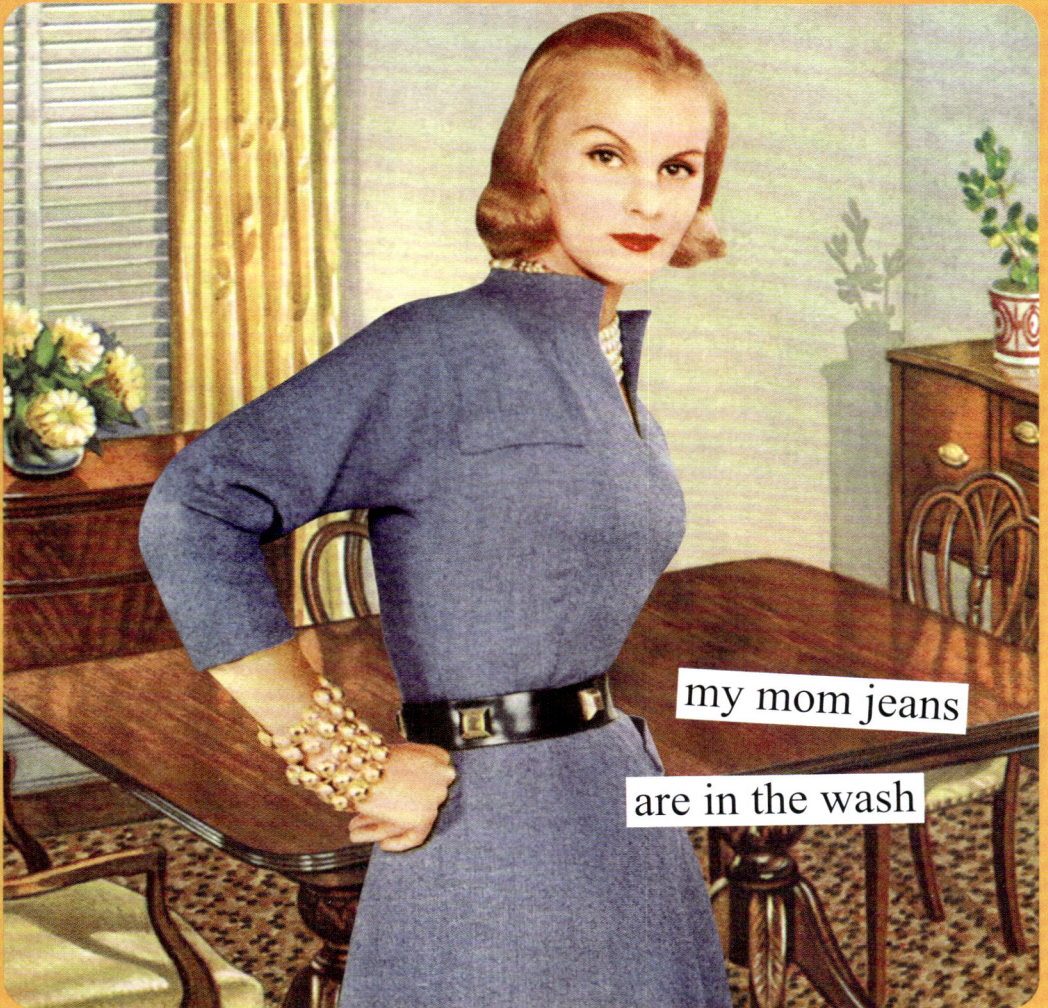

my mom jeans are in the wash

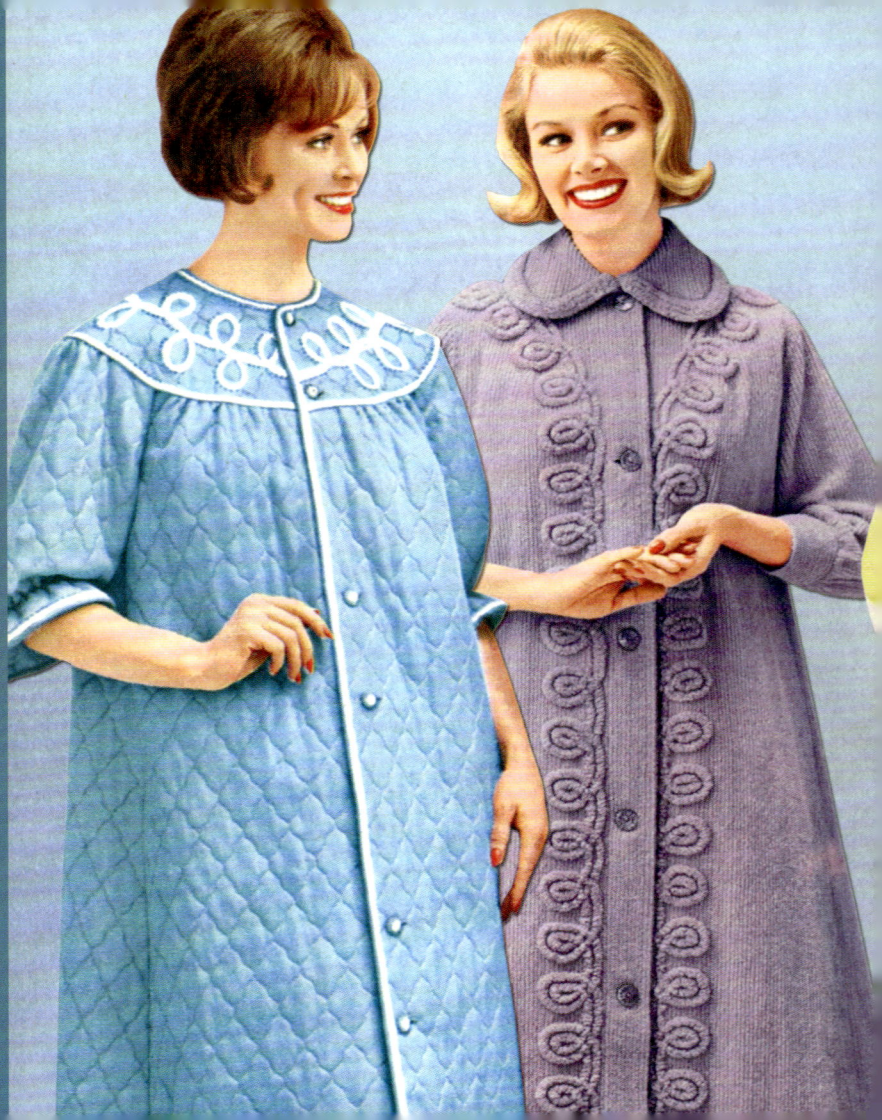

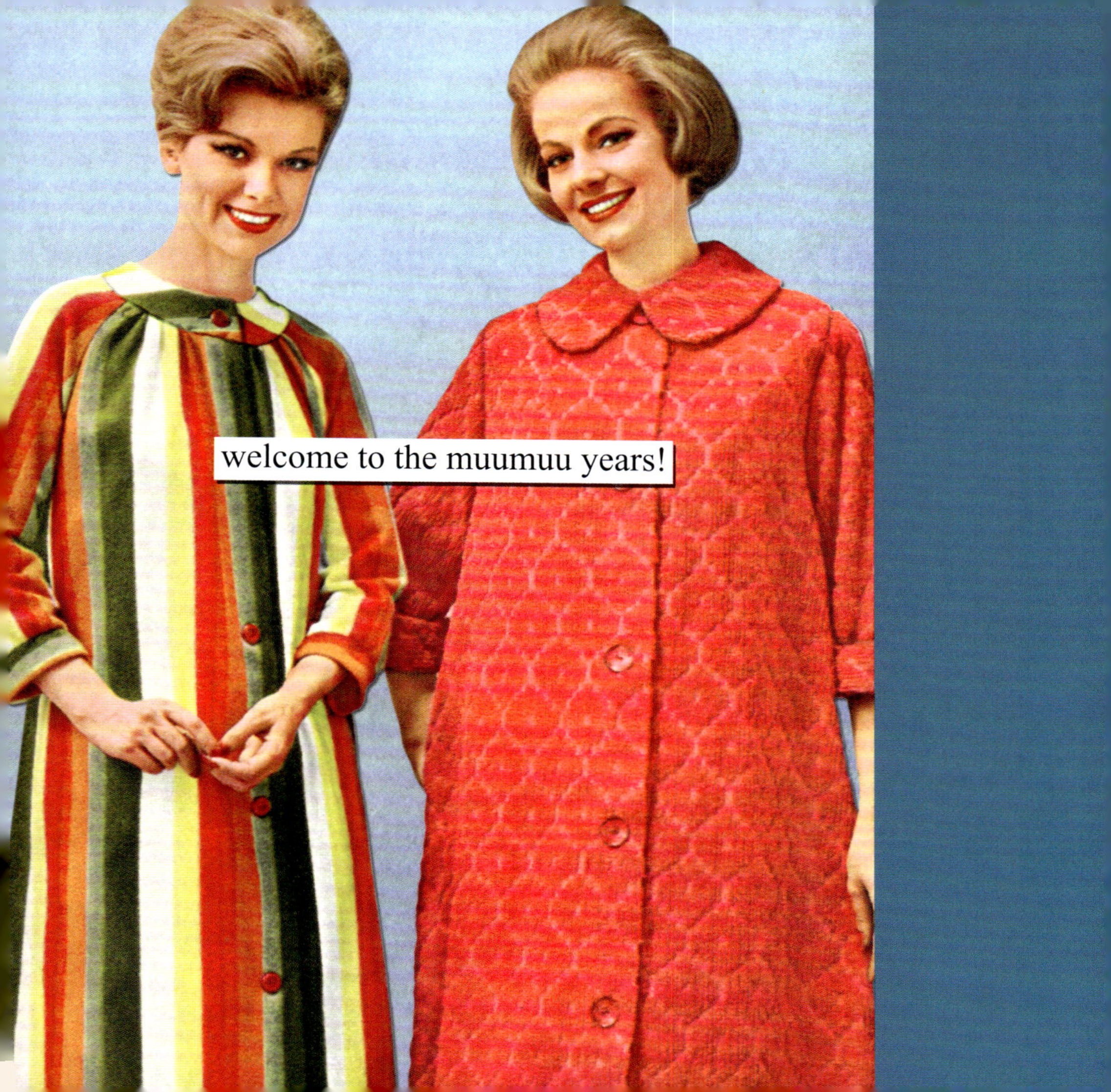

welcome to the muumuu years!

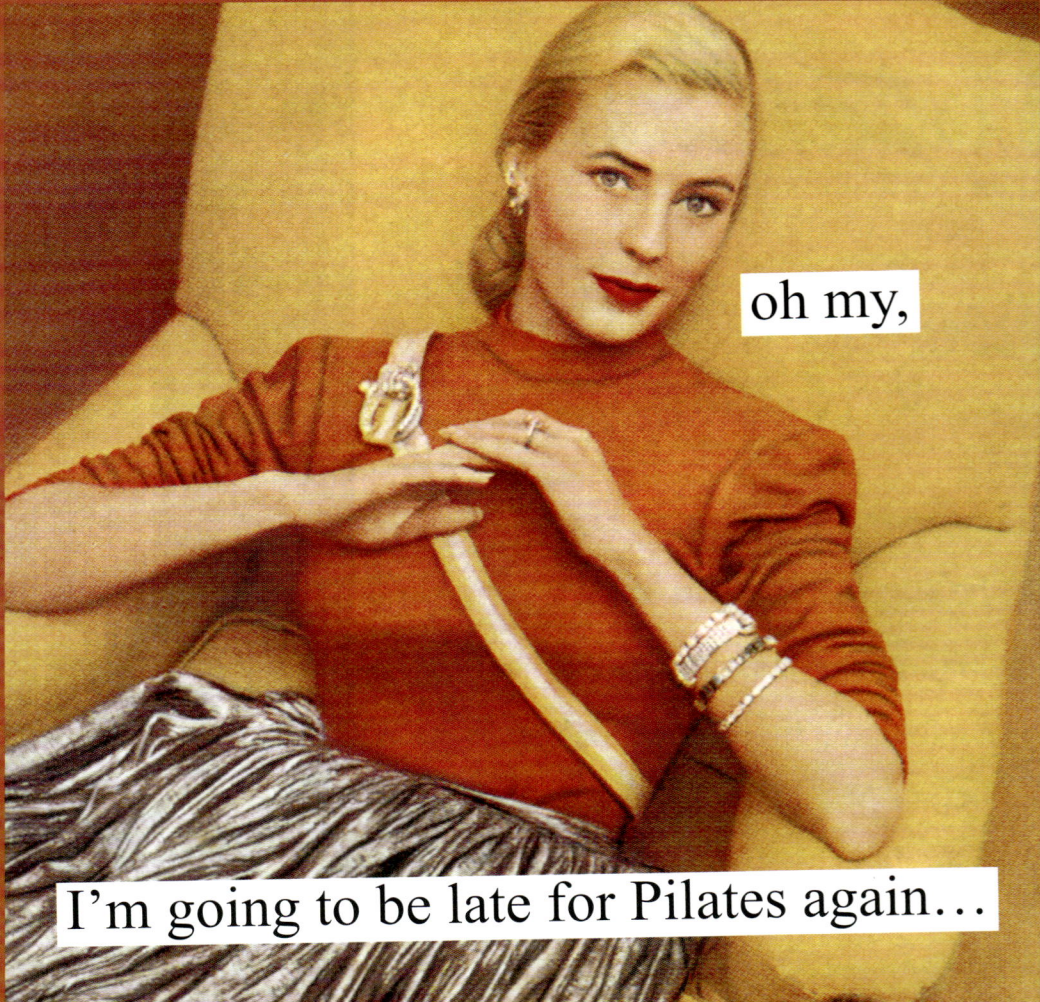

oh my,

I'm going to be late for Pilates again...

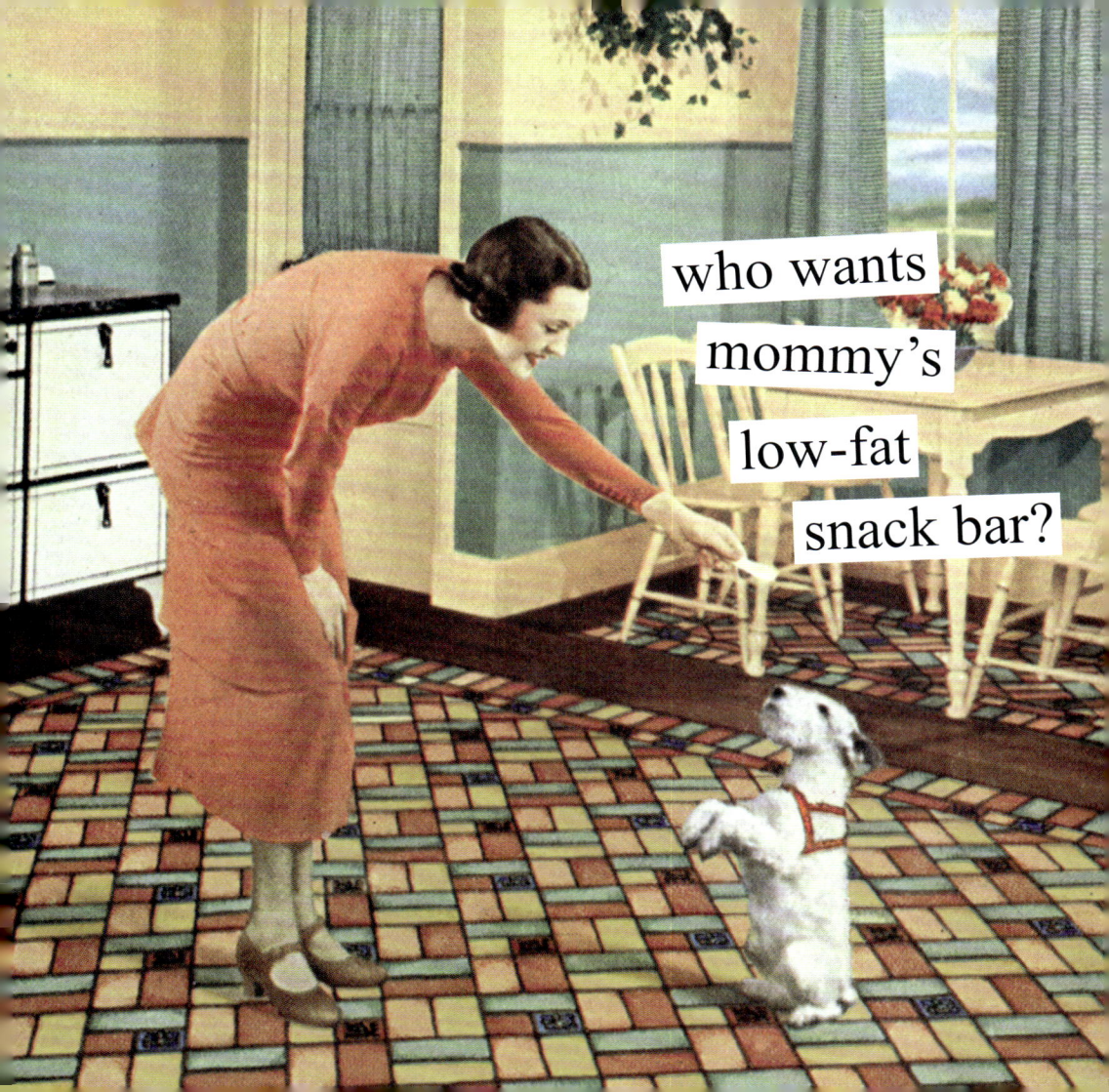

who wants mommy's low-fat snack bar?

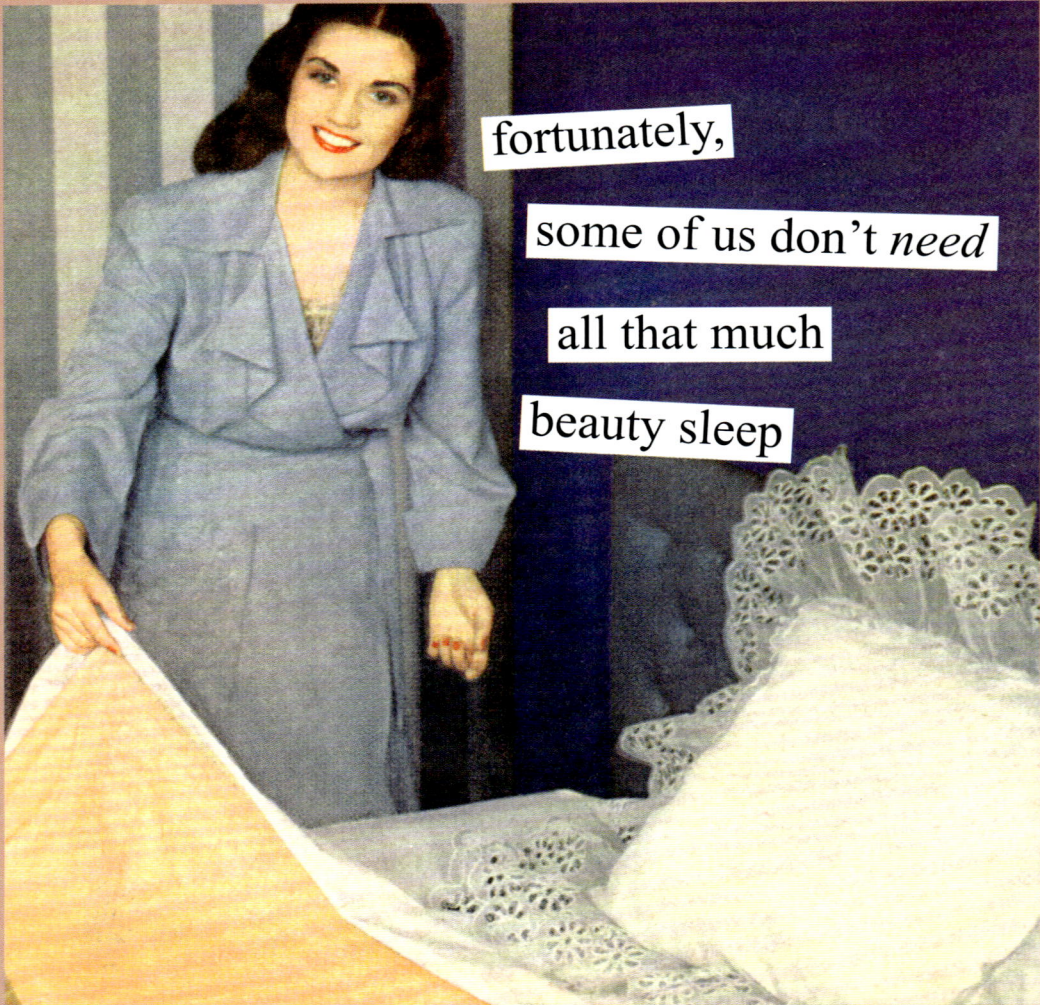

I believe the word you're searching for is "divine"

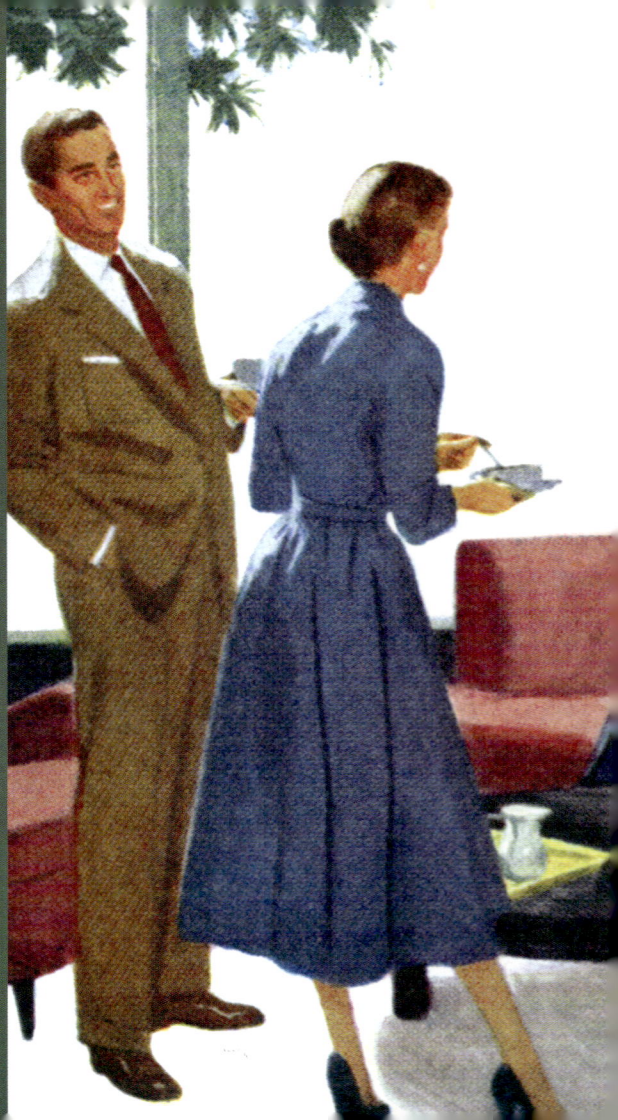

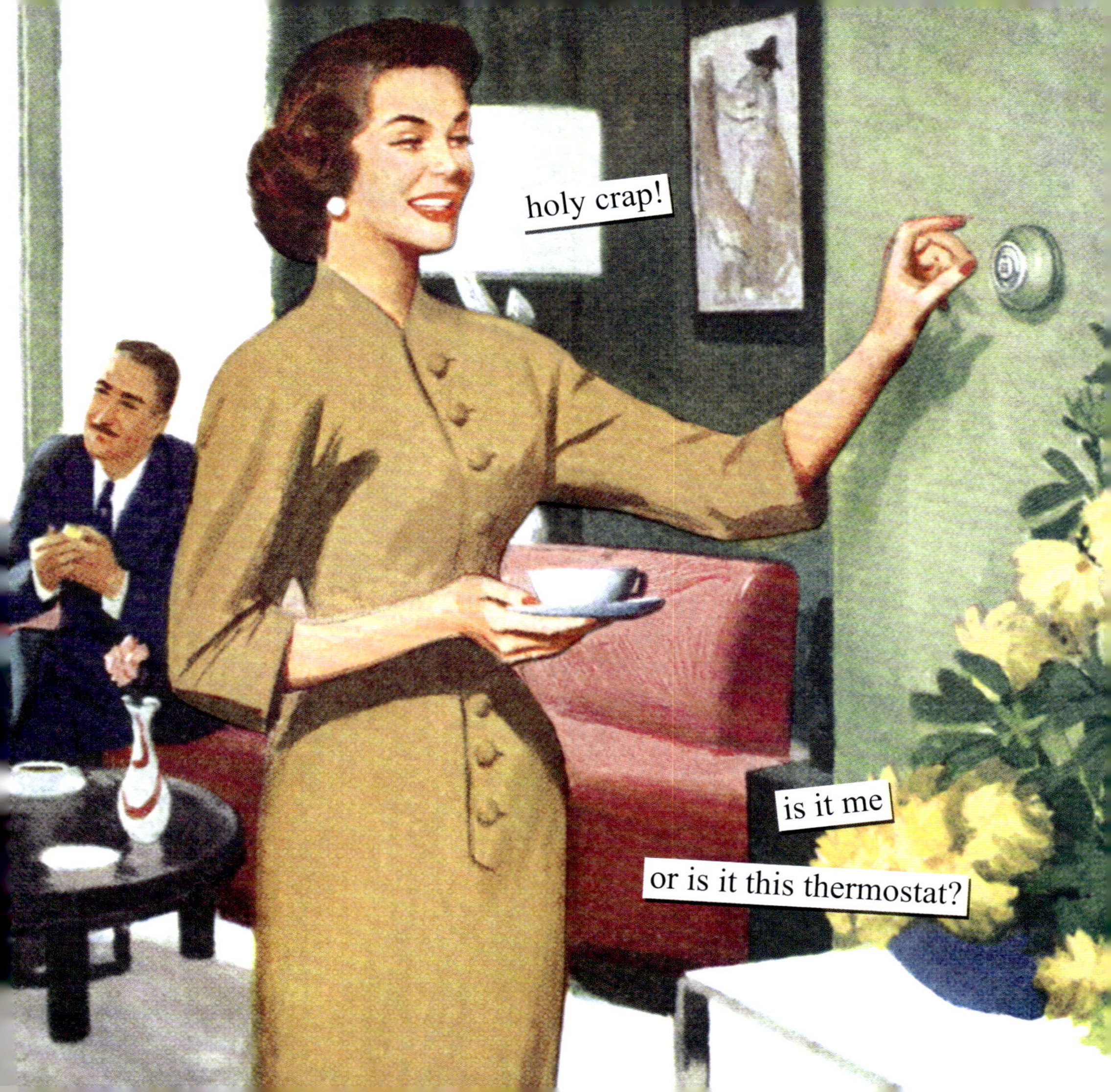
holy crap!
is it me
or is it this thermostat?

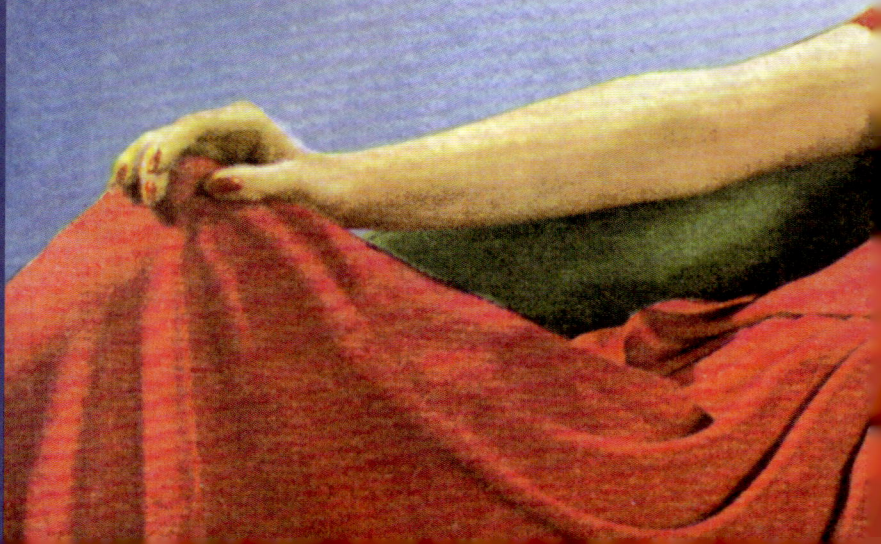

Let me know

when they invent

Cool Yoga.

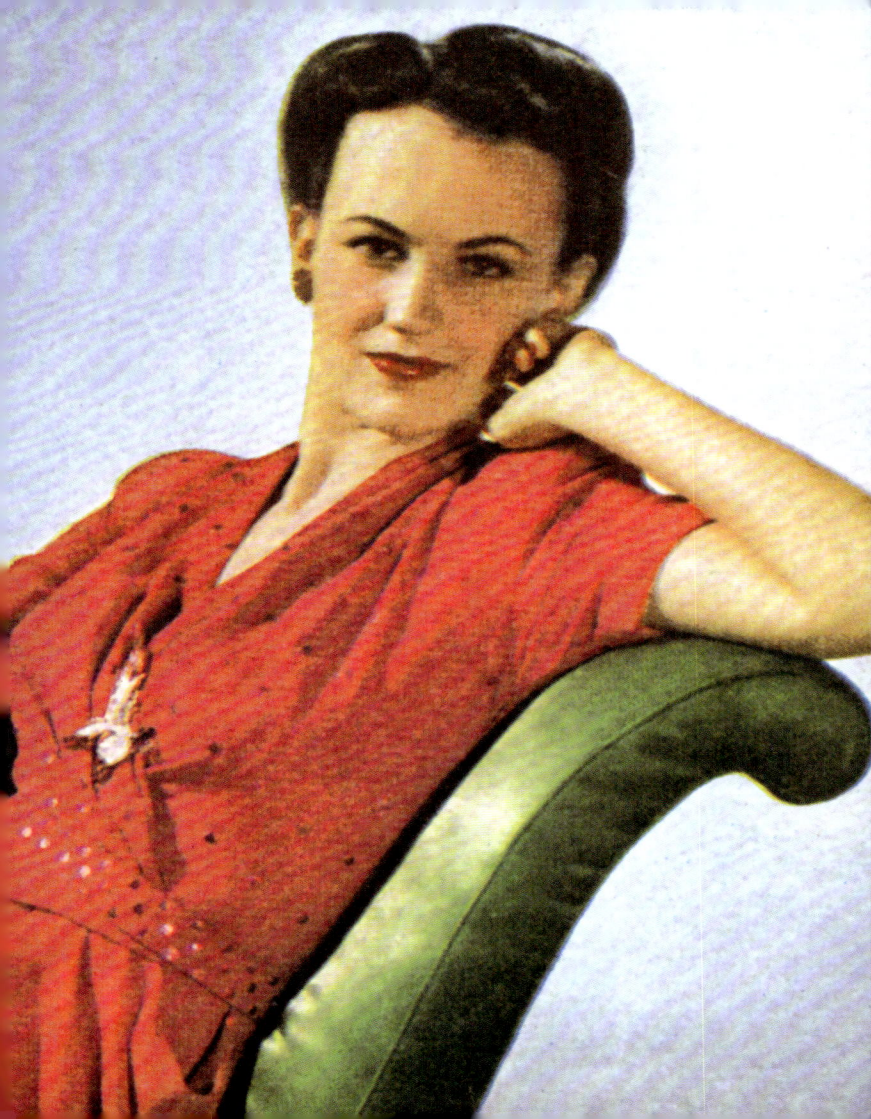

please call back

when I

give a damn

she was

comforted

by the

knowledge

that

they were

helpless without her

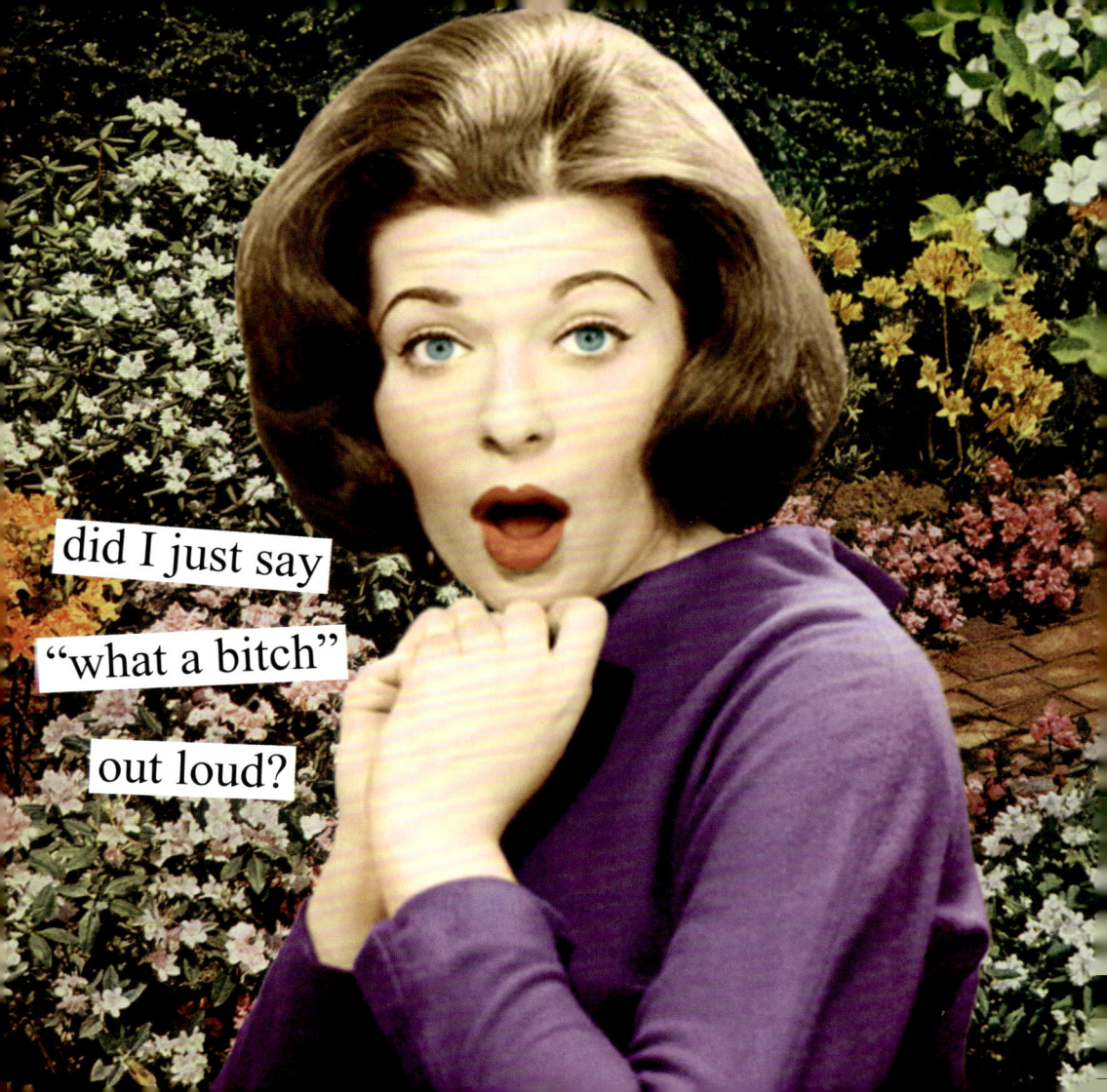

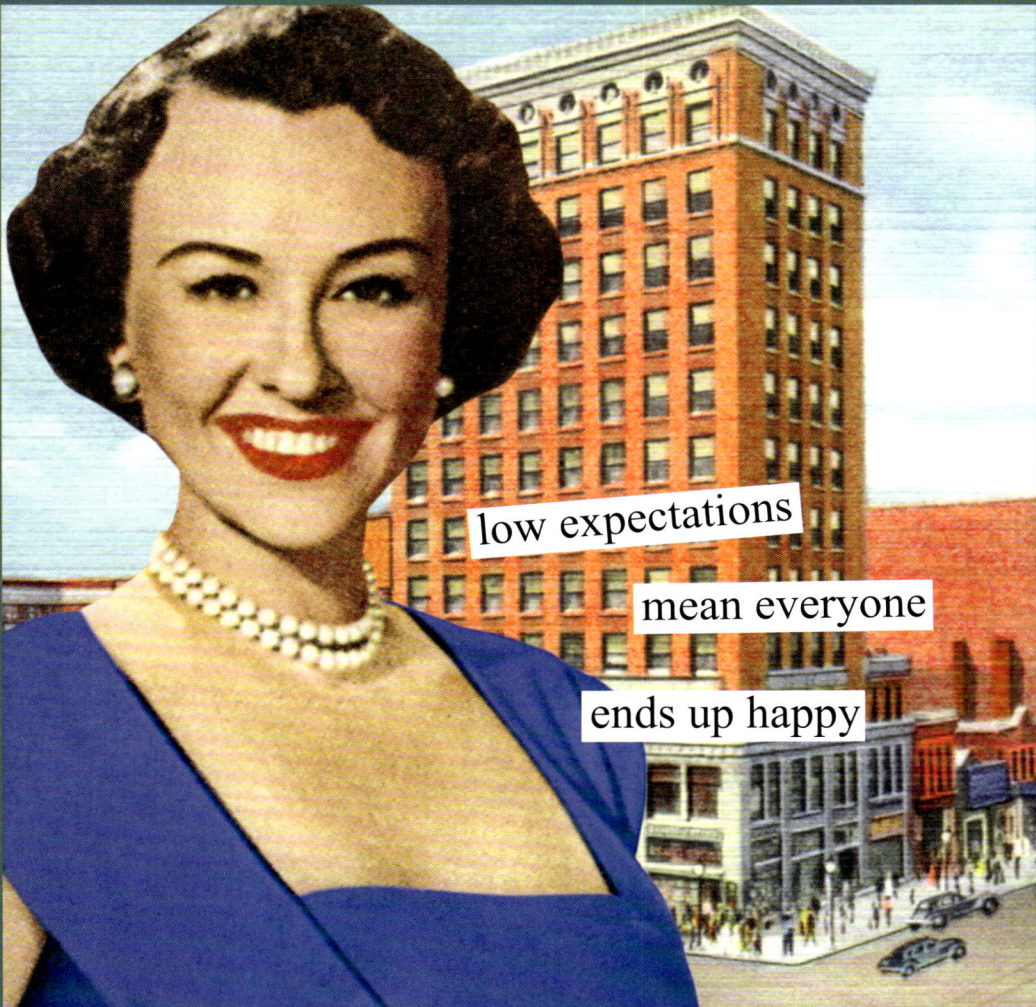

low expectations mean everyone ends up happy

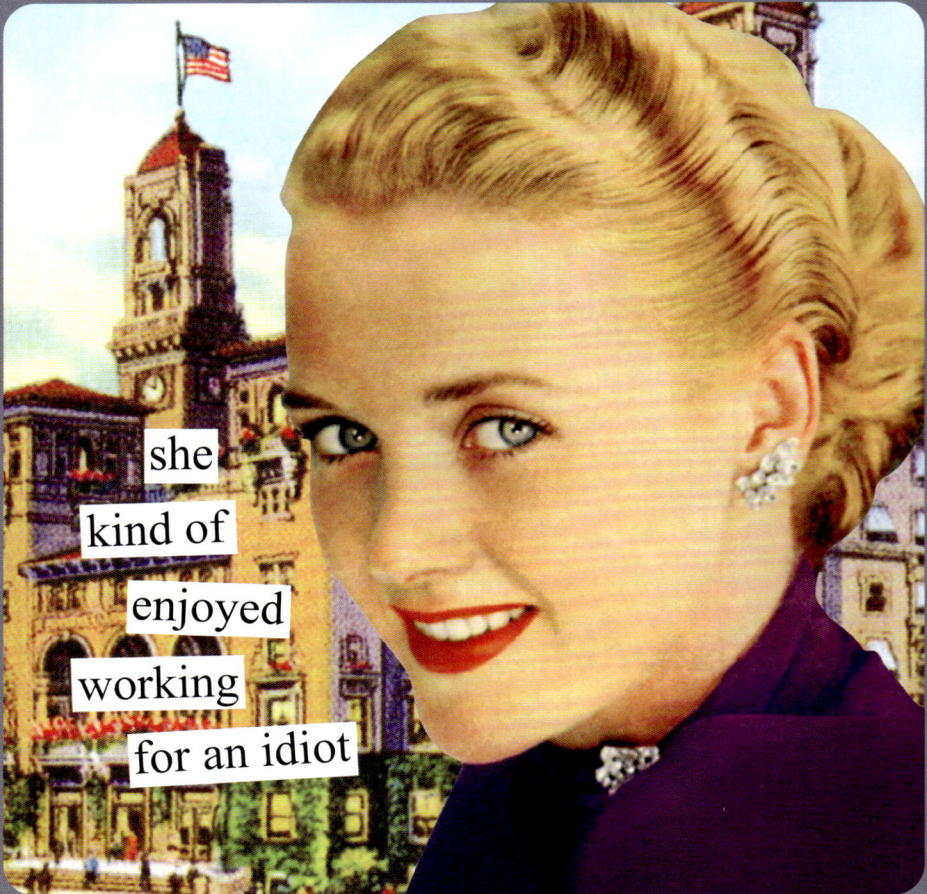

she
kind of
enjoyed
working
for an idiot

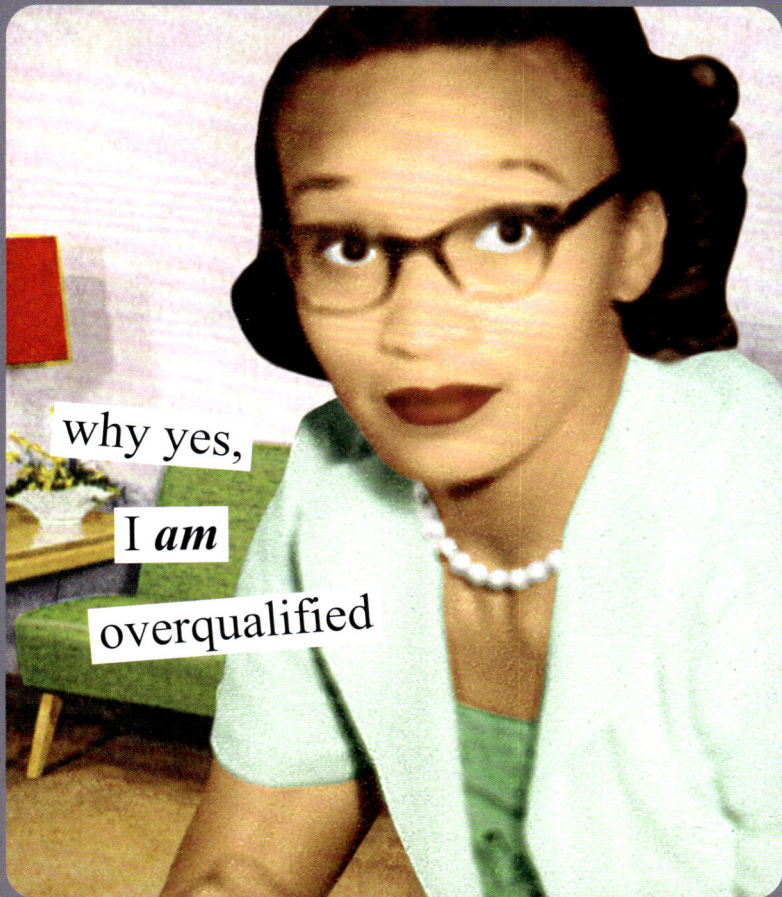

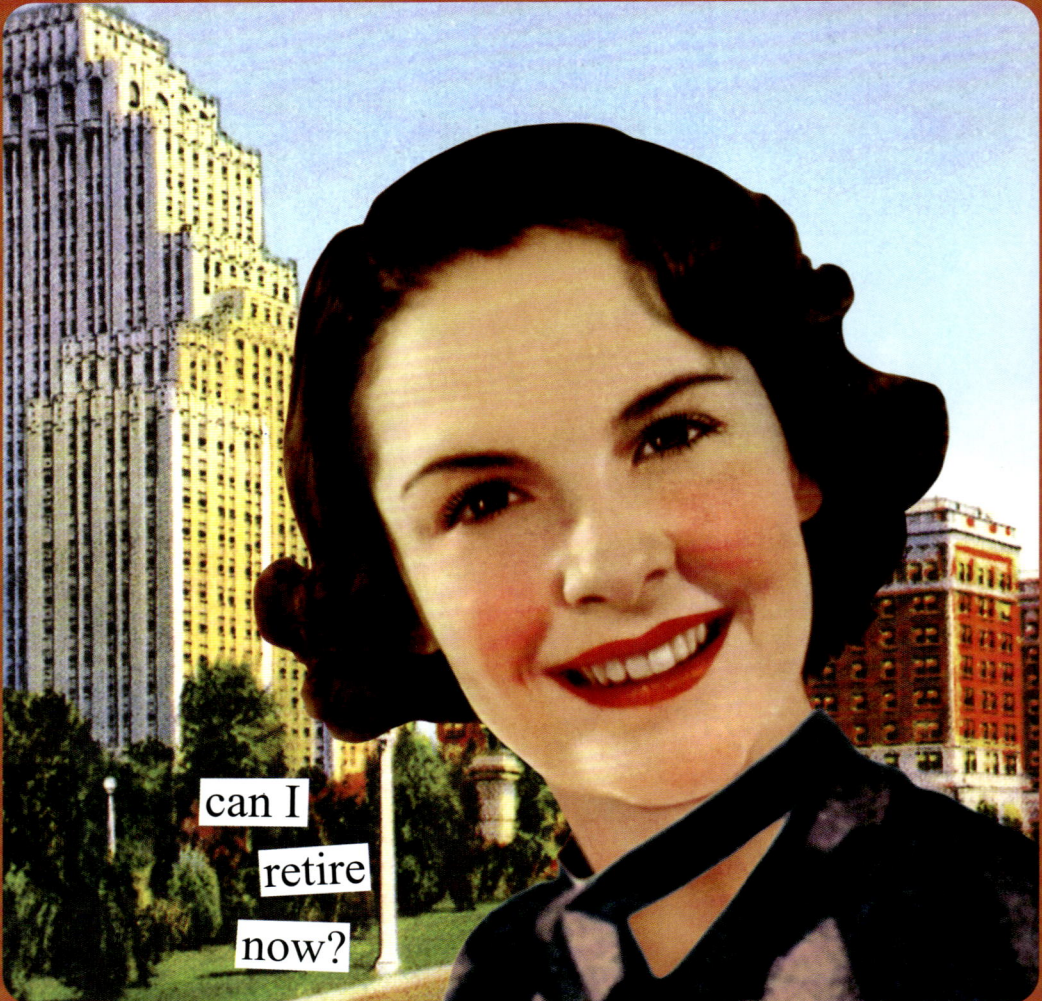

can I
retire
now?

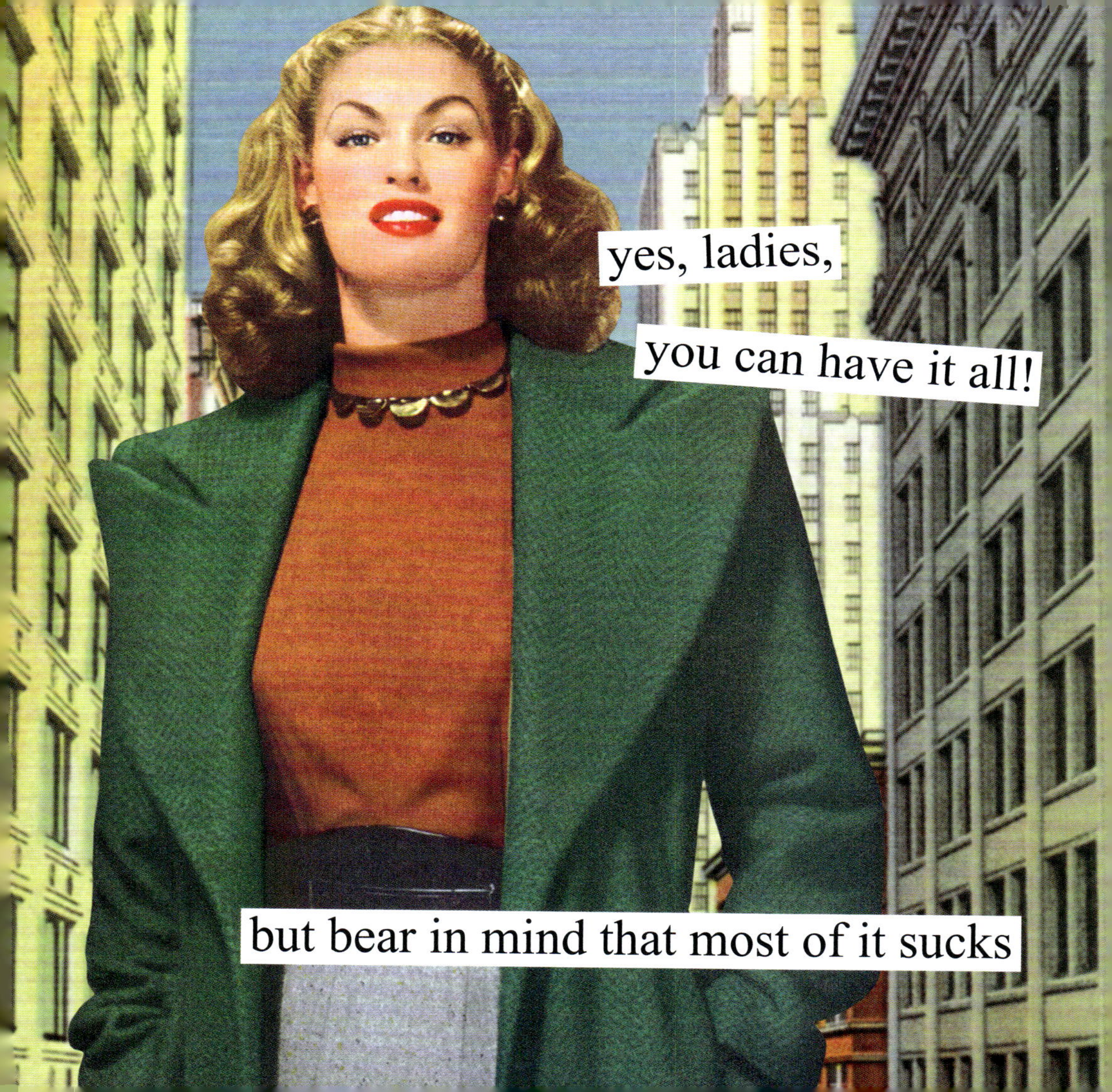
yes, ladies,
you can have it all!
but bear in mind that most of it sucks

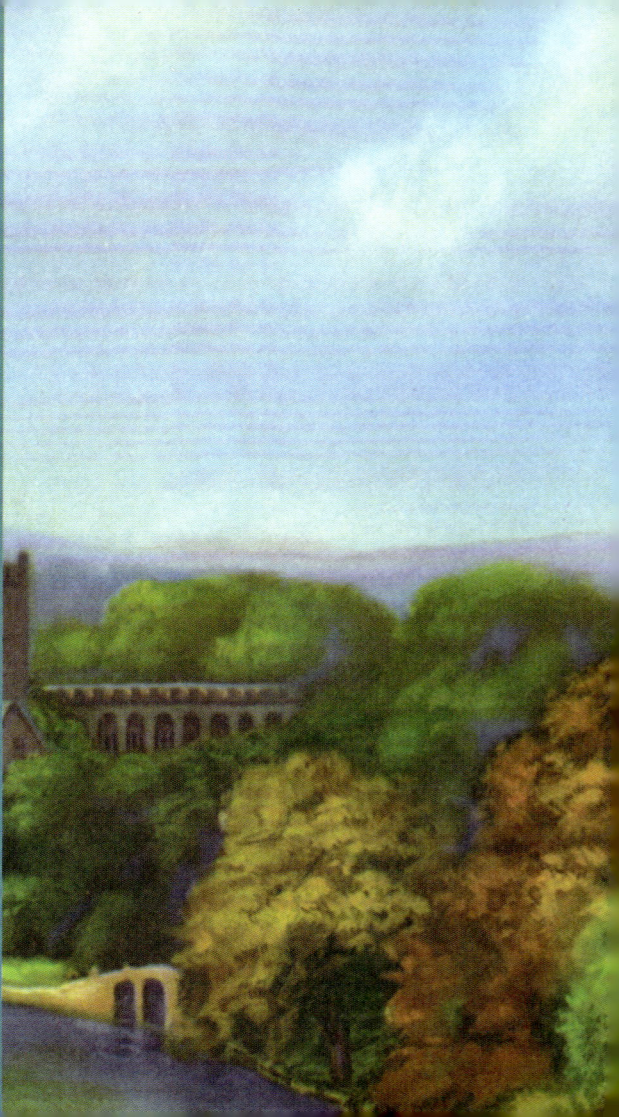

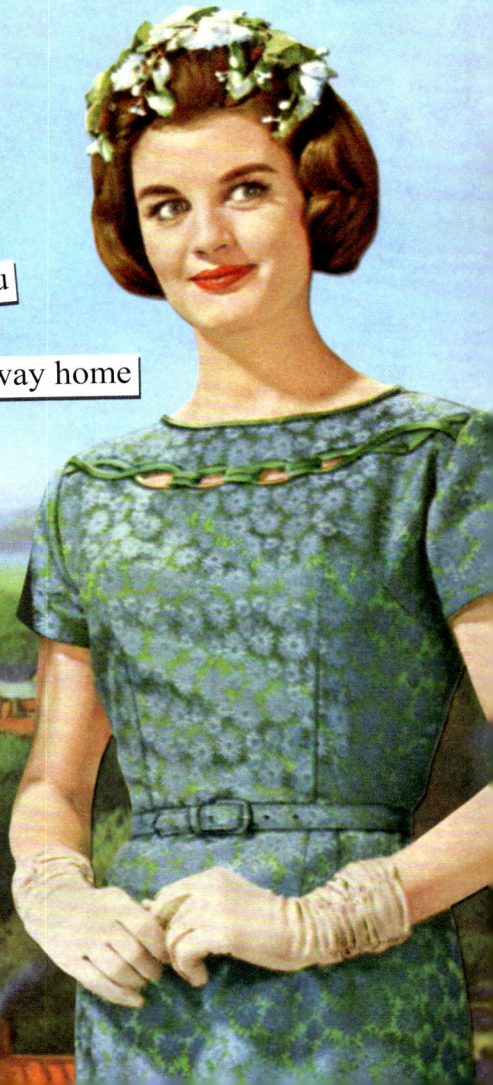

a birthday

is just nature's way

of reminding you

to pick up wine on the way home

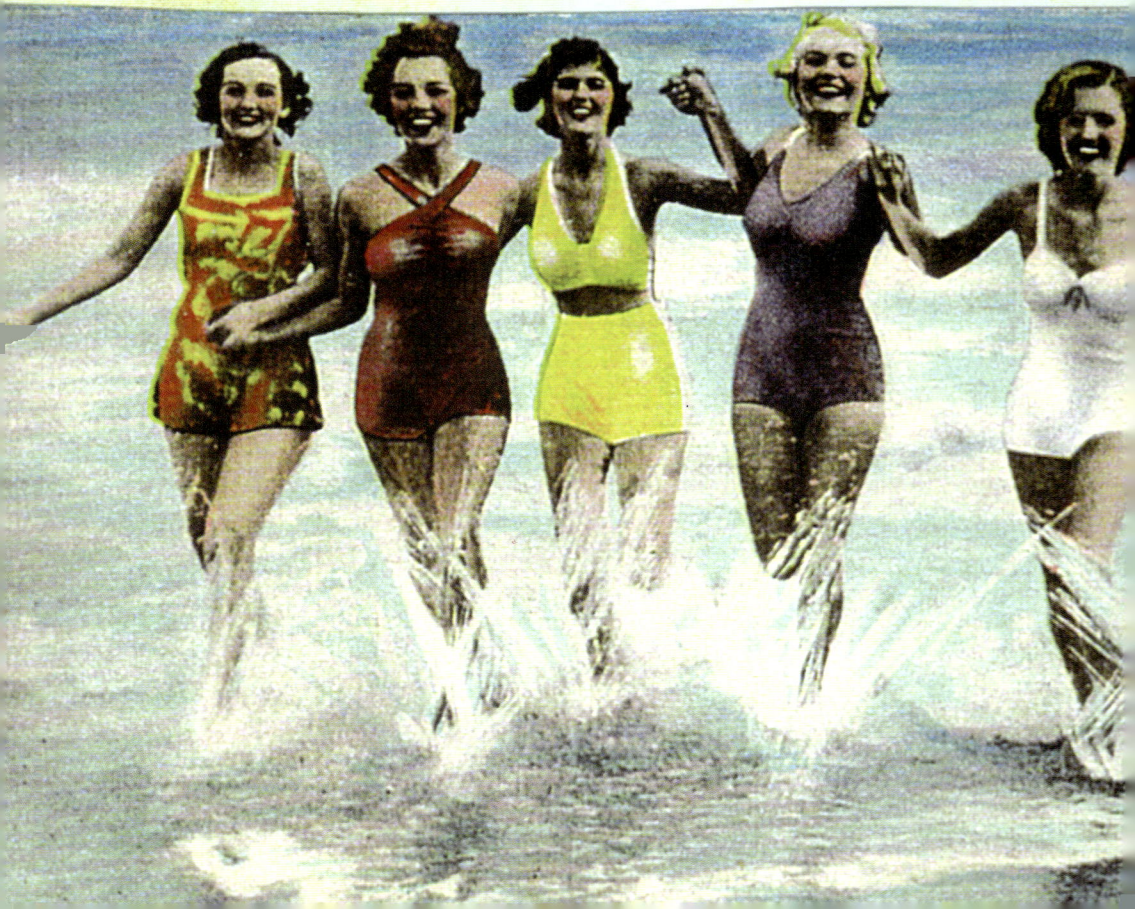
born to be wild

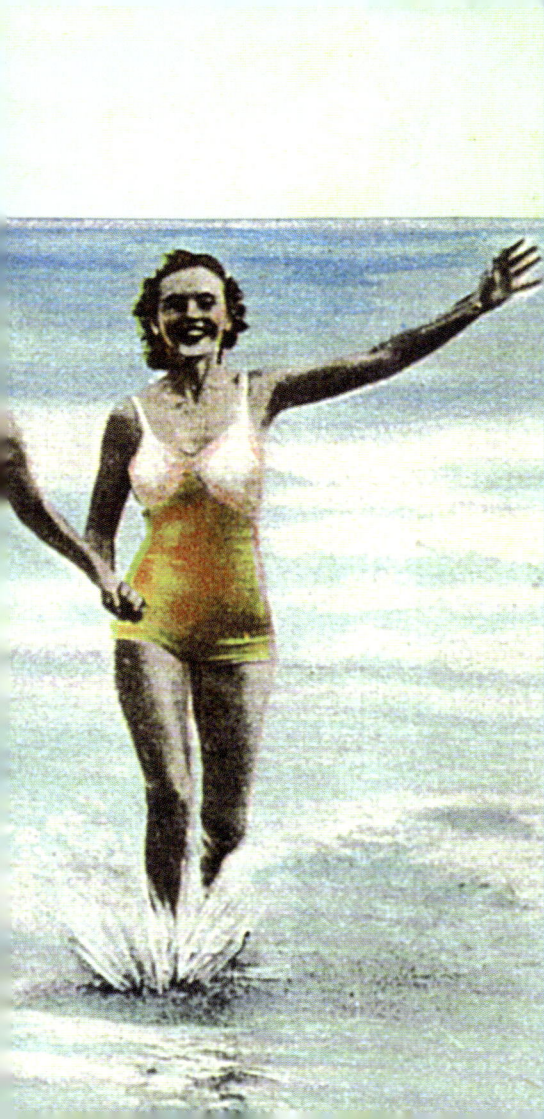

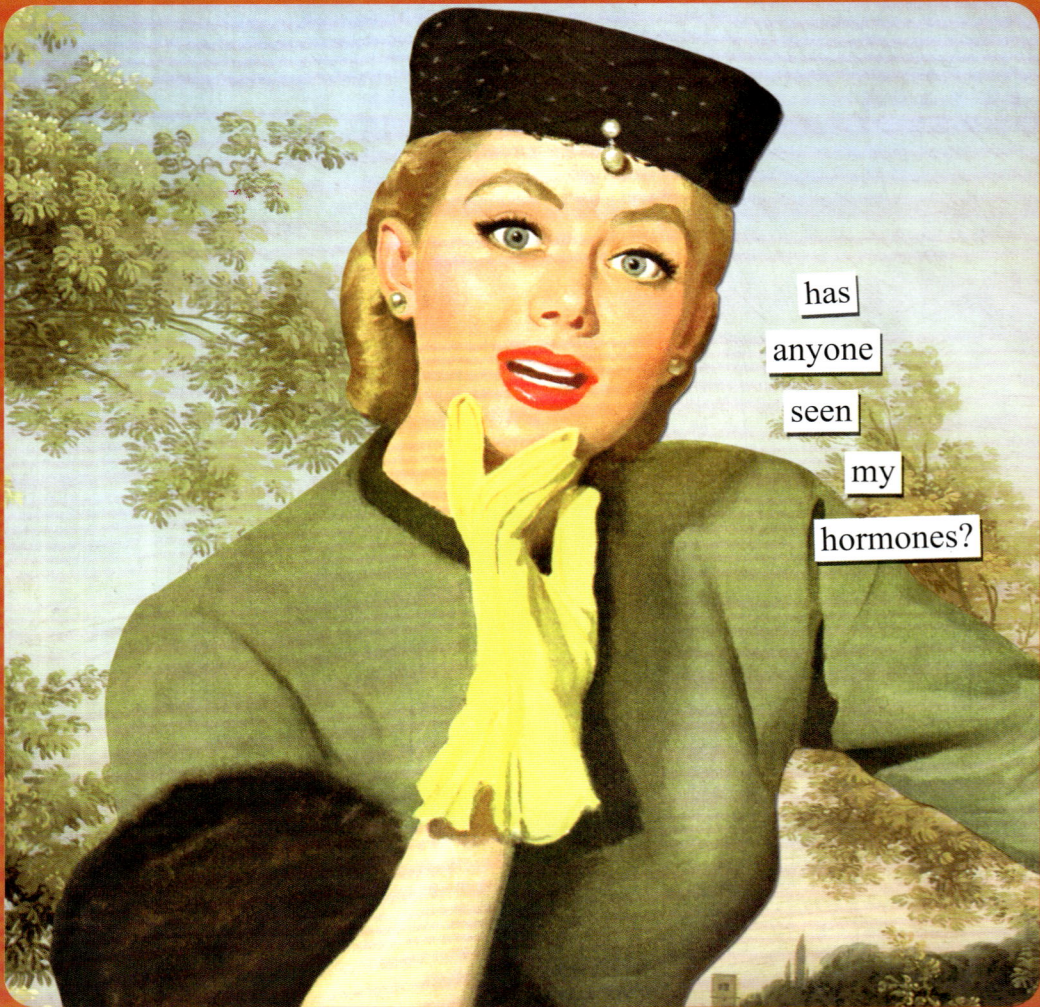

has
anyone
seen
my
hormones?

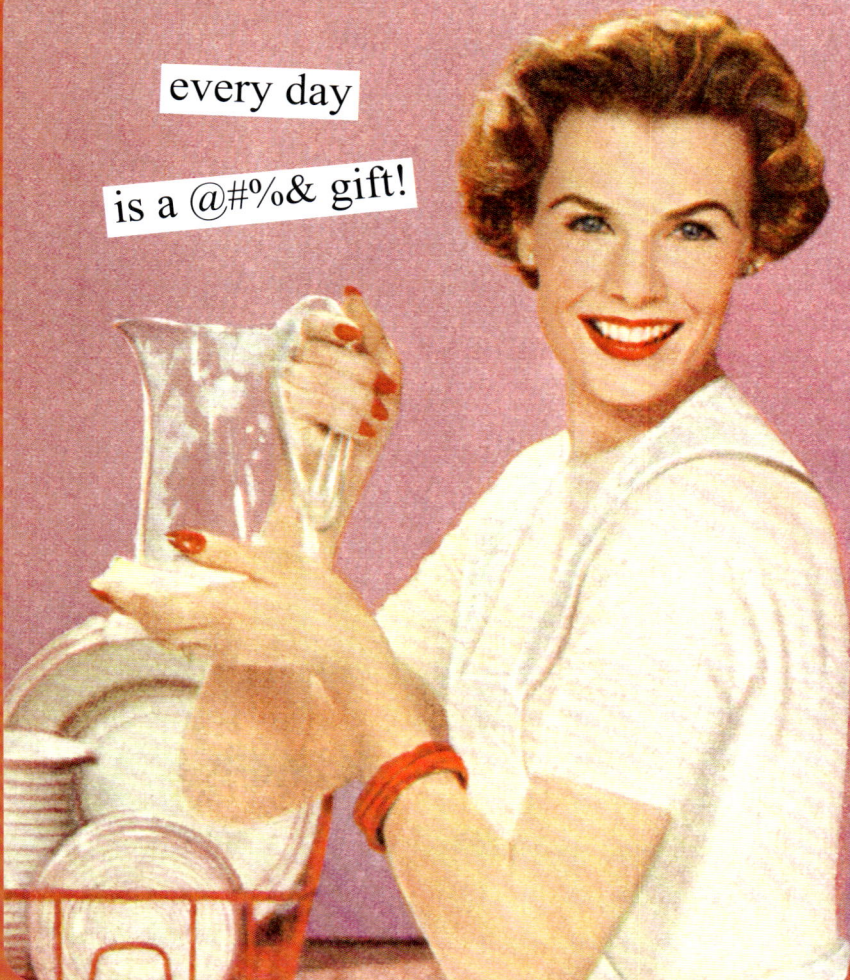

every day

is a @#%& gift!

they'd been married so long

he was almost beginning to make sense

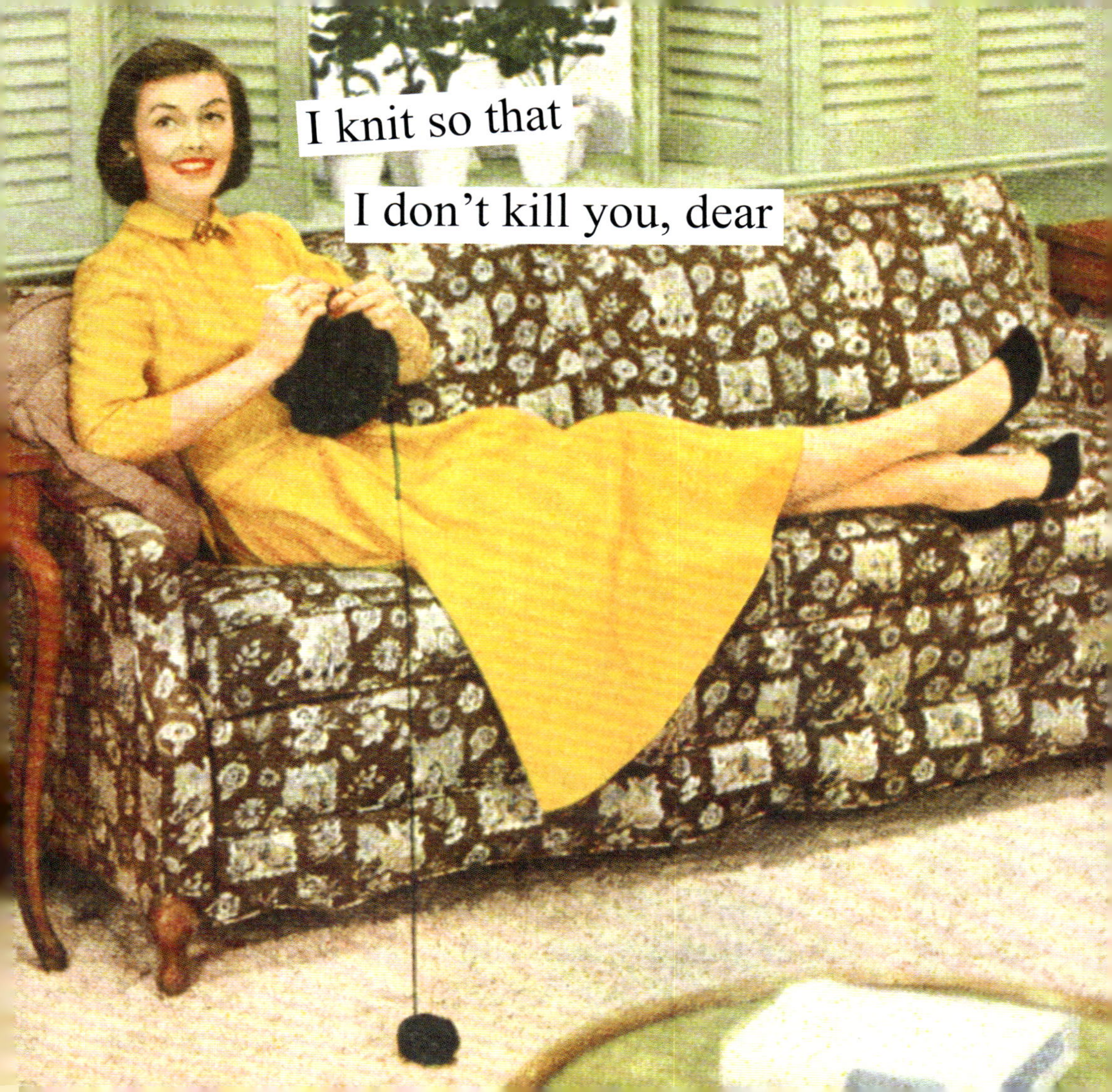
I knit so that
I don’t kill you, dear

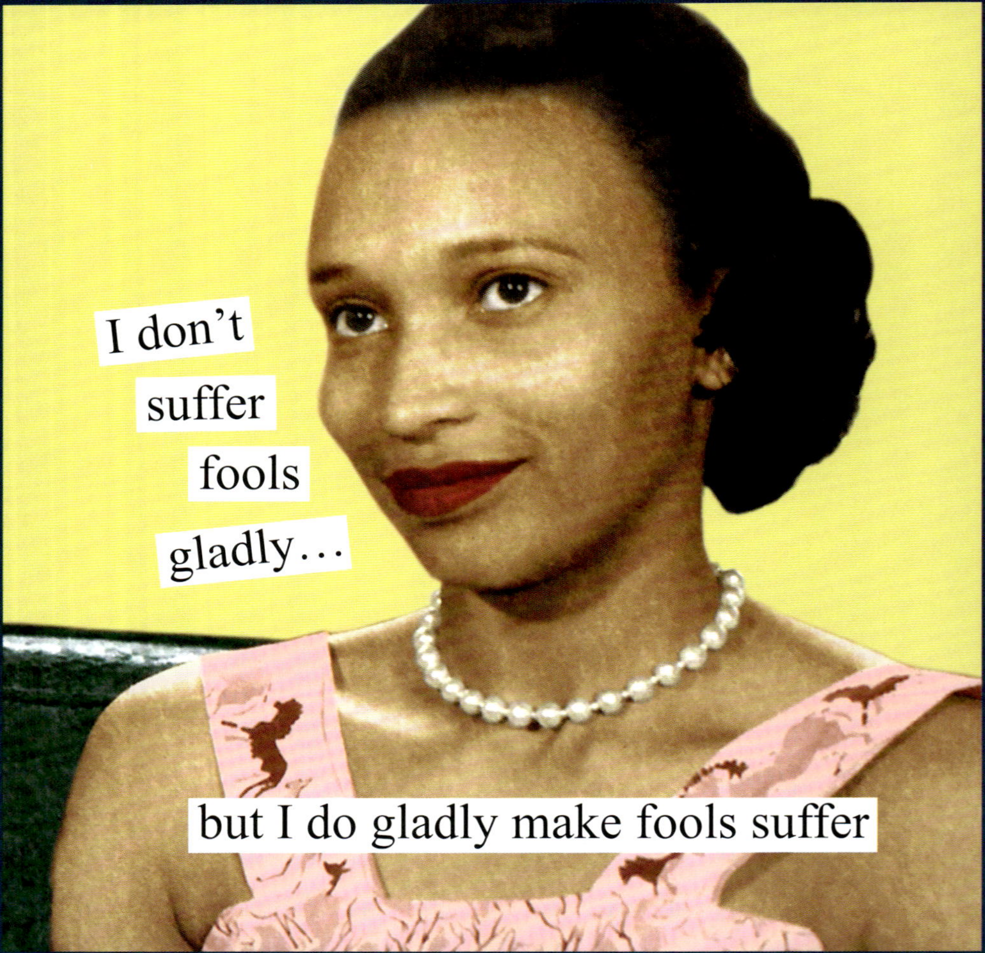
I don't
suffer
fools
gladly…
but I do gladly make fools suffer

I
don't
believe
I've *ever* had
too much fun

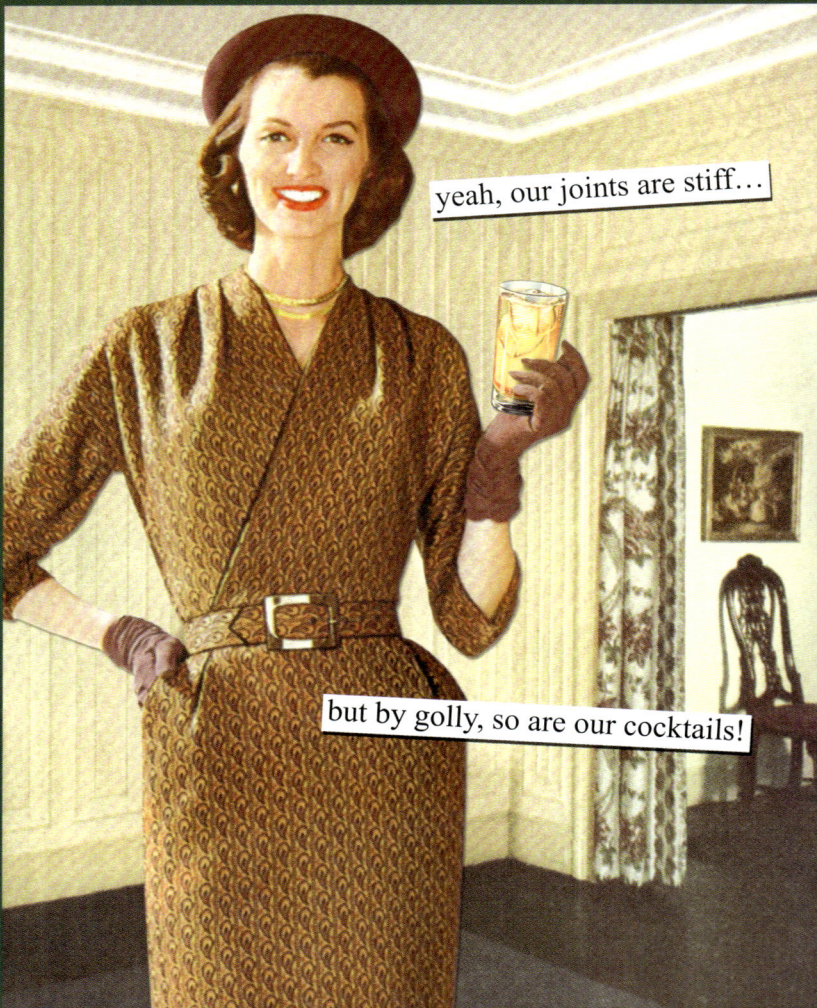

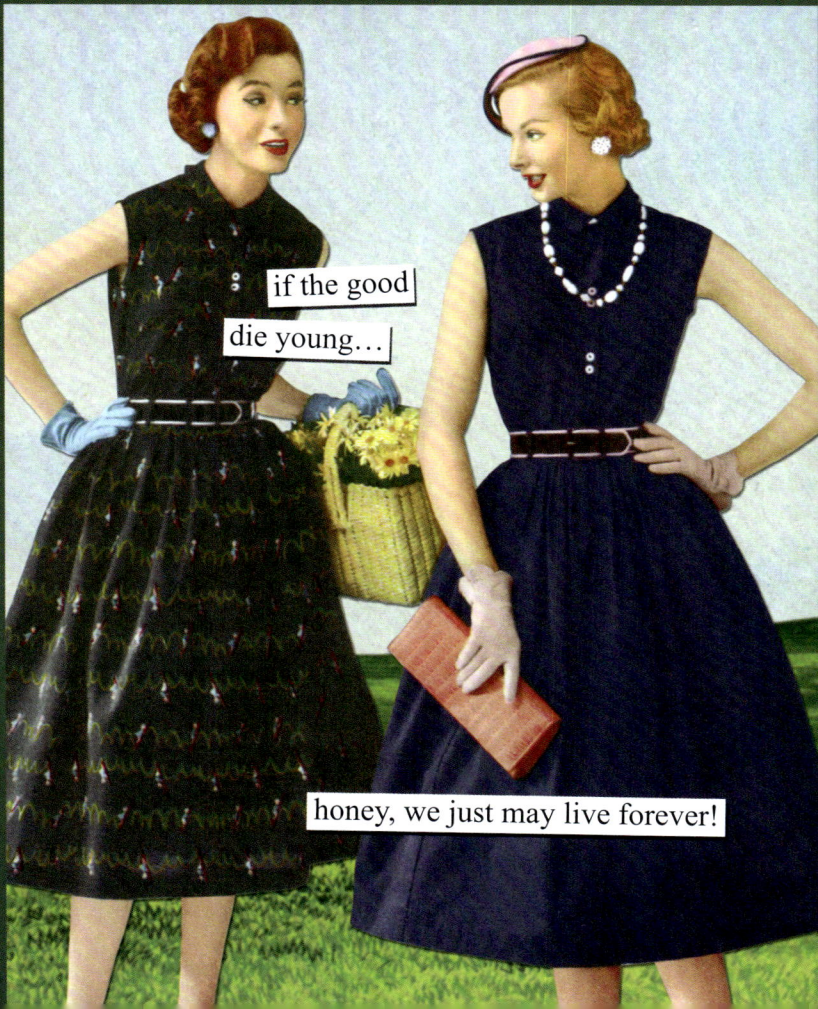

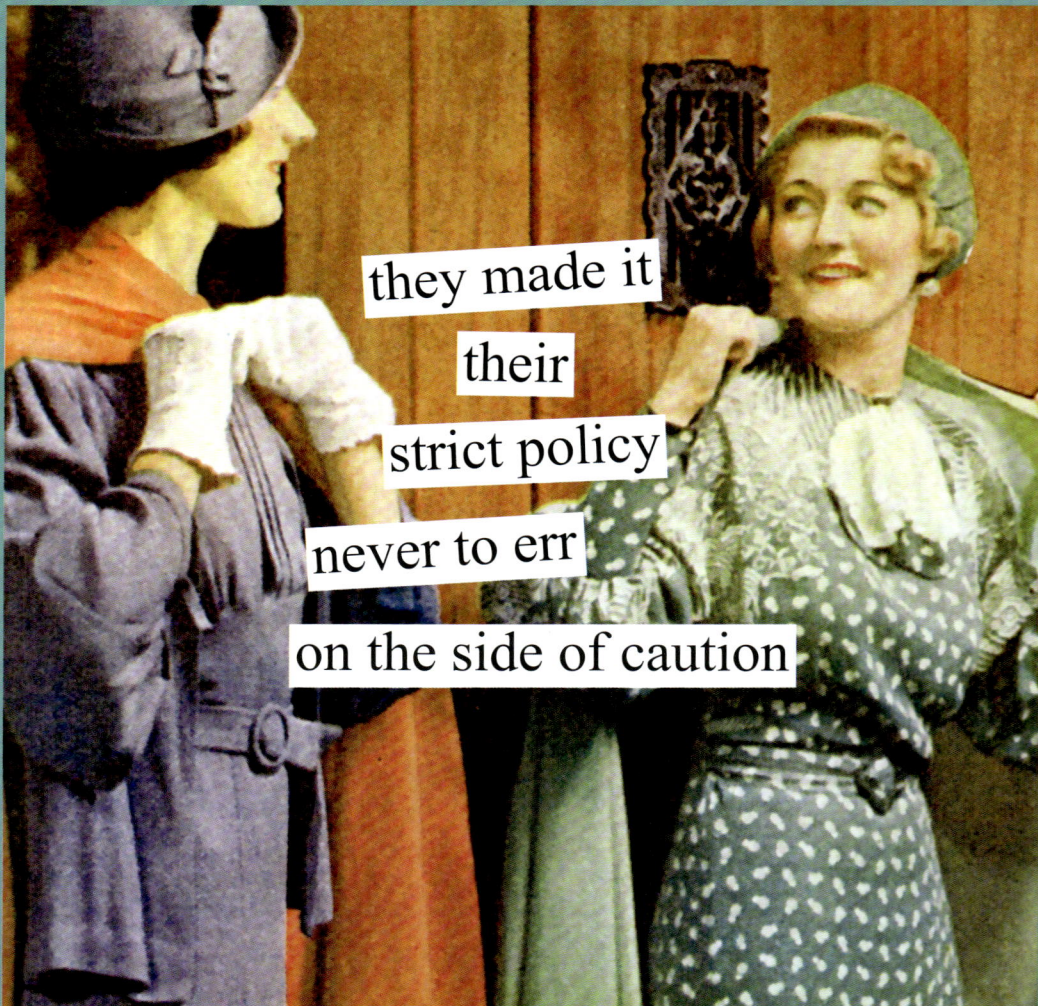

they made it
their
strict policy
never to err
on the side of caution

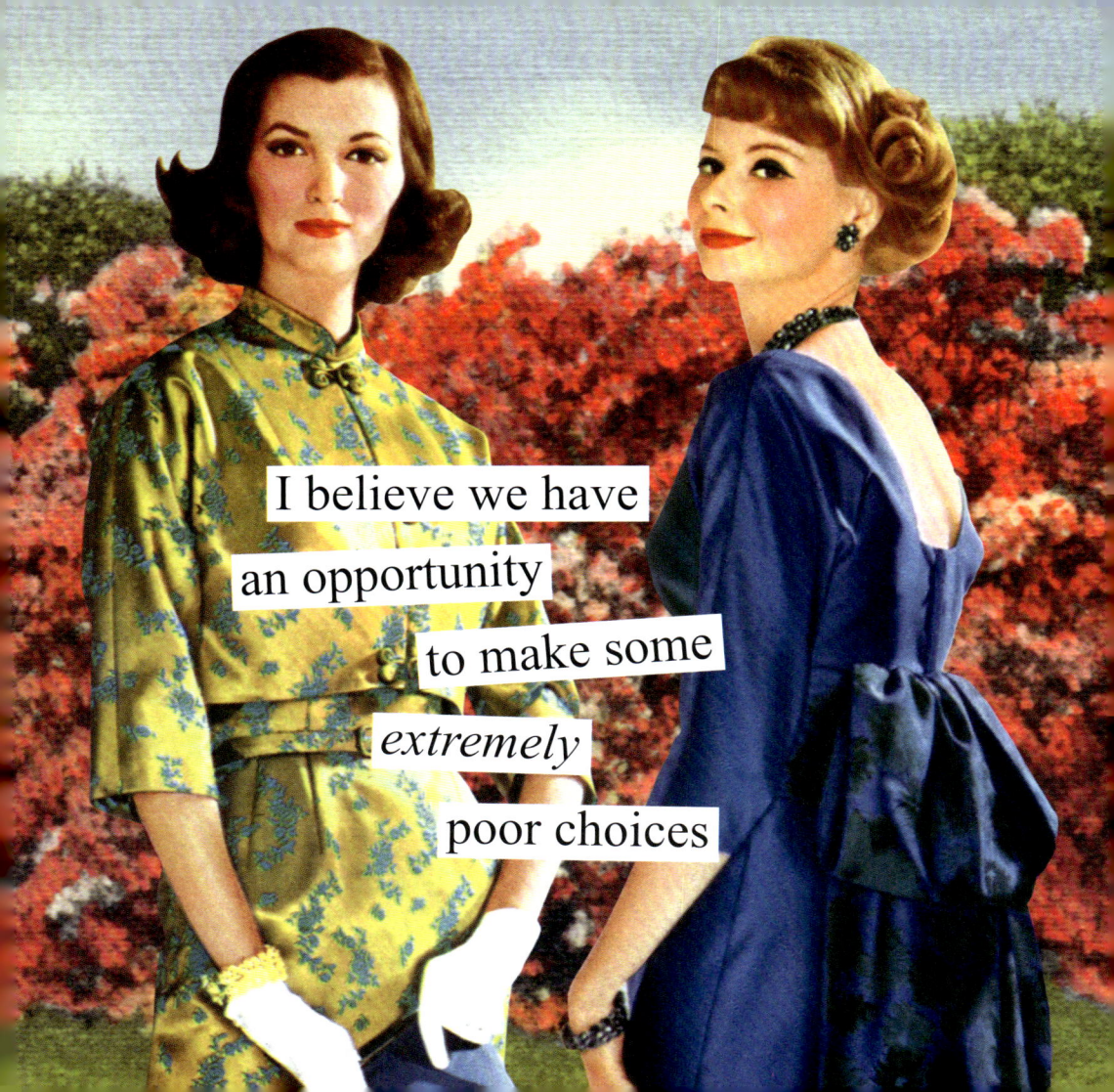

I believe we have an opportunity to make some *extremely* poor choices

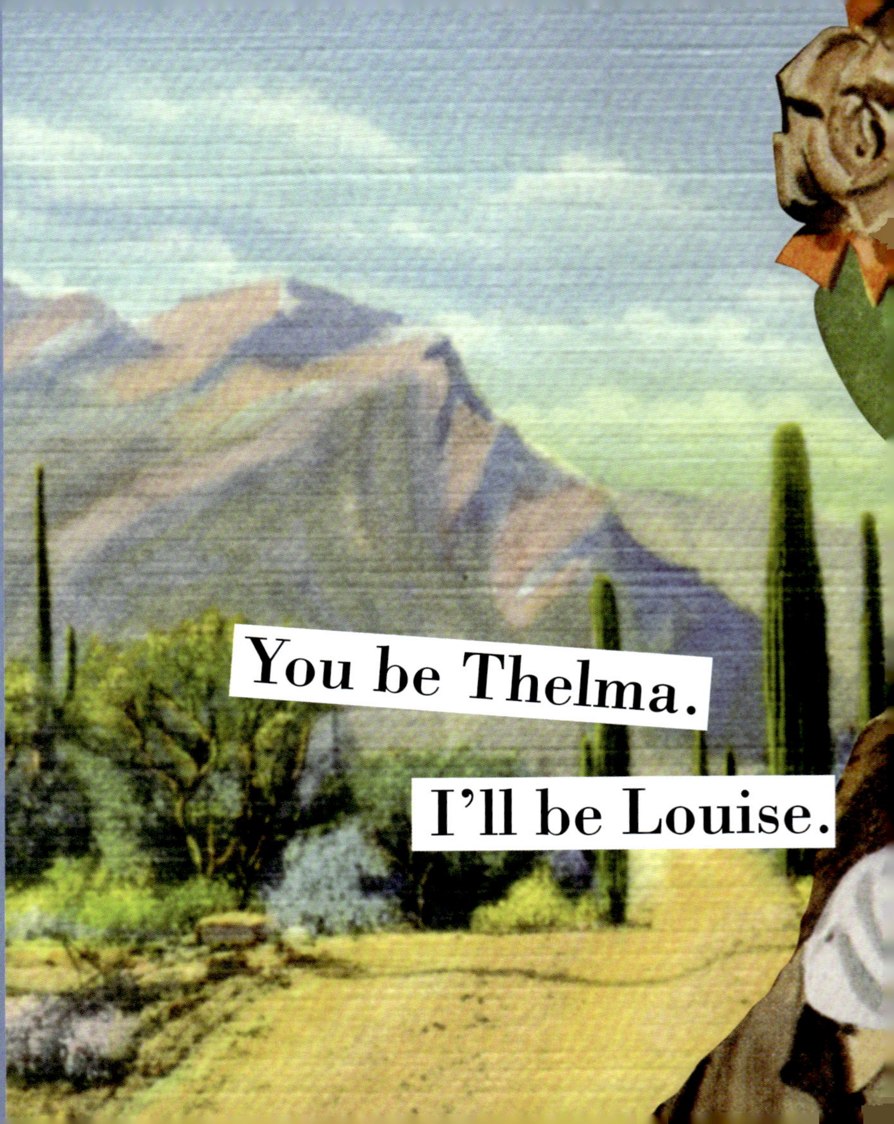

You be Thelma.

I'll be Louise.

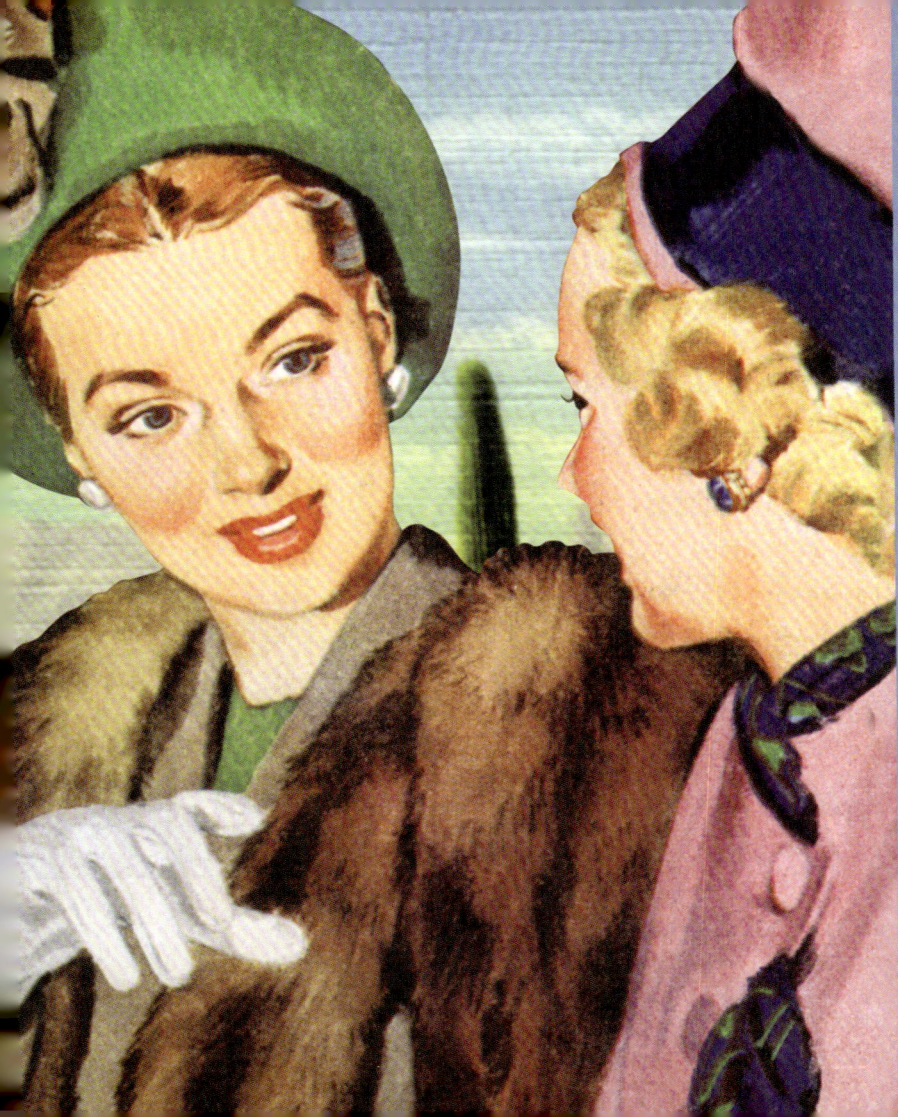

I wish

this were

gin

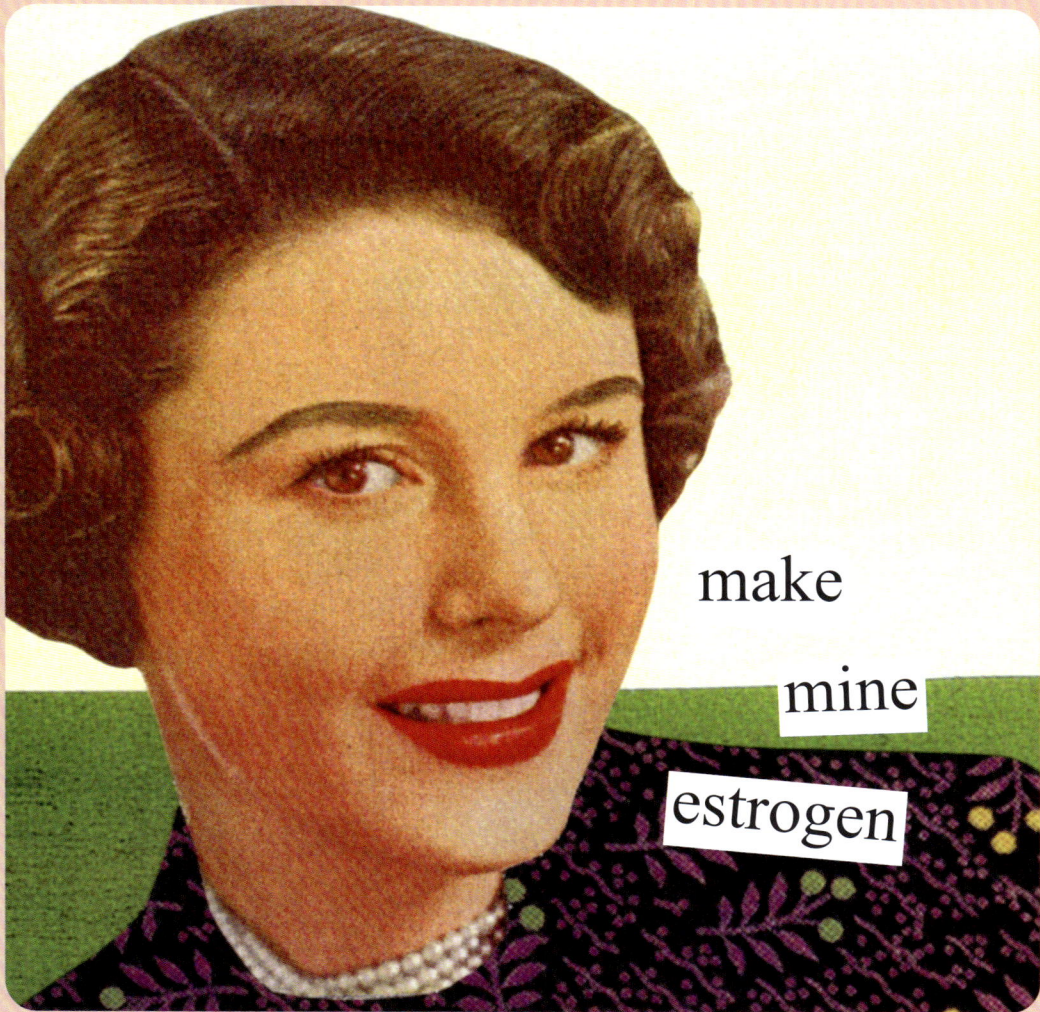

make

mine

estrogen

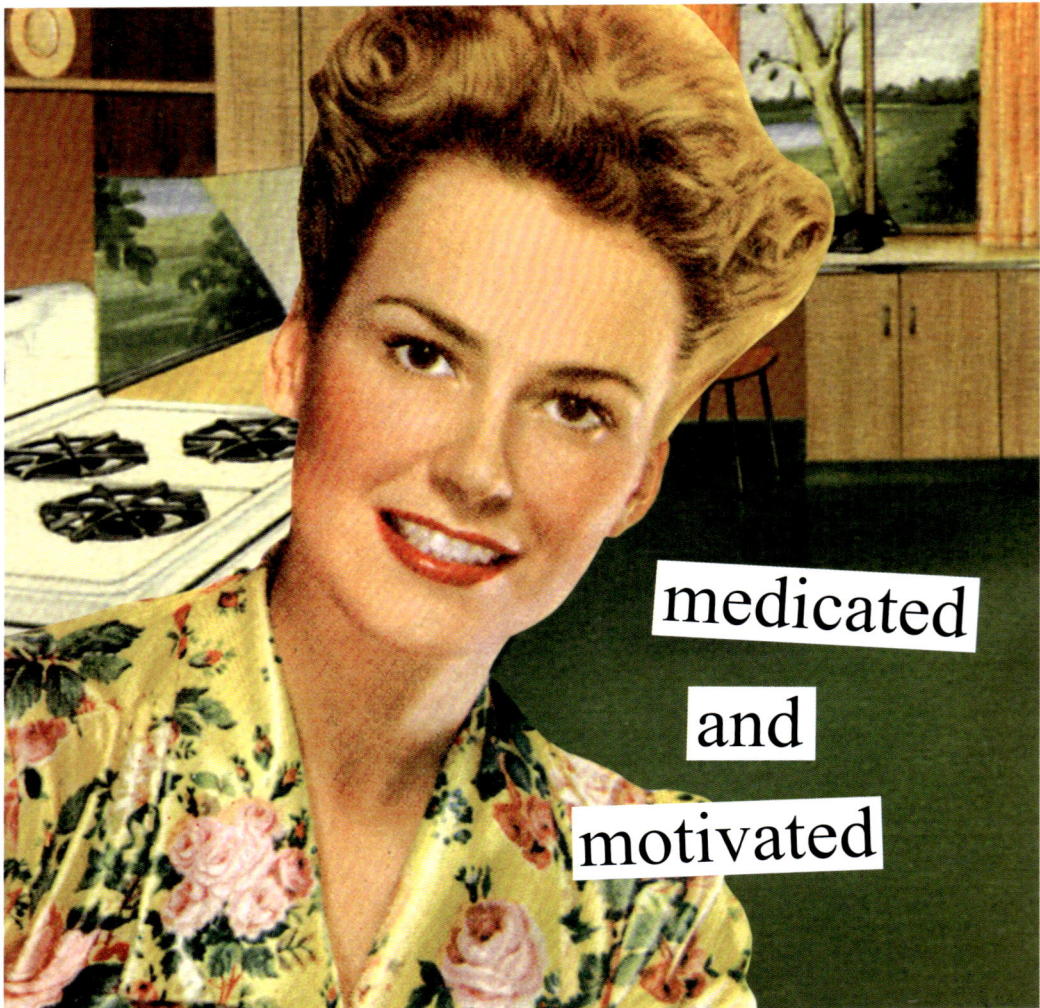

medicated

and

motivated

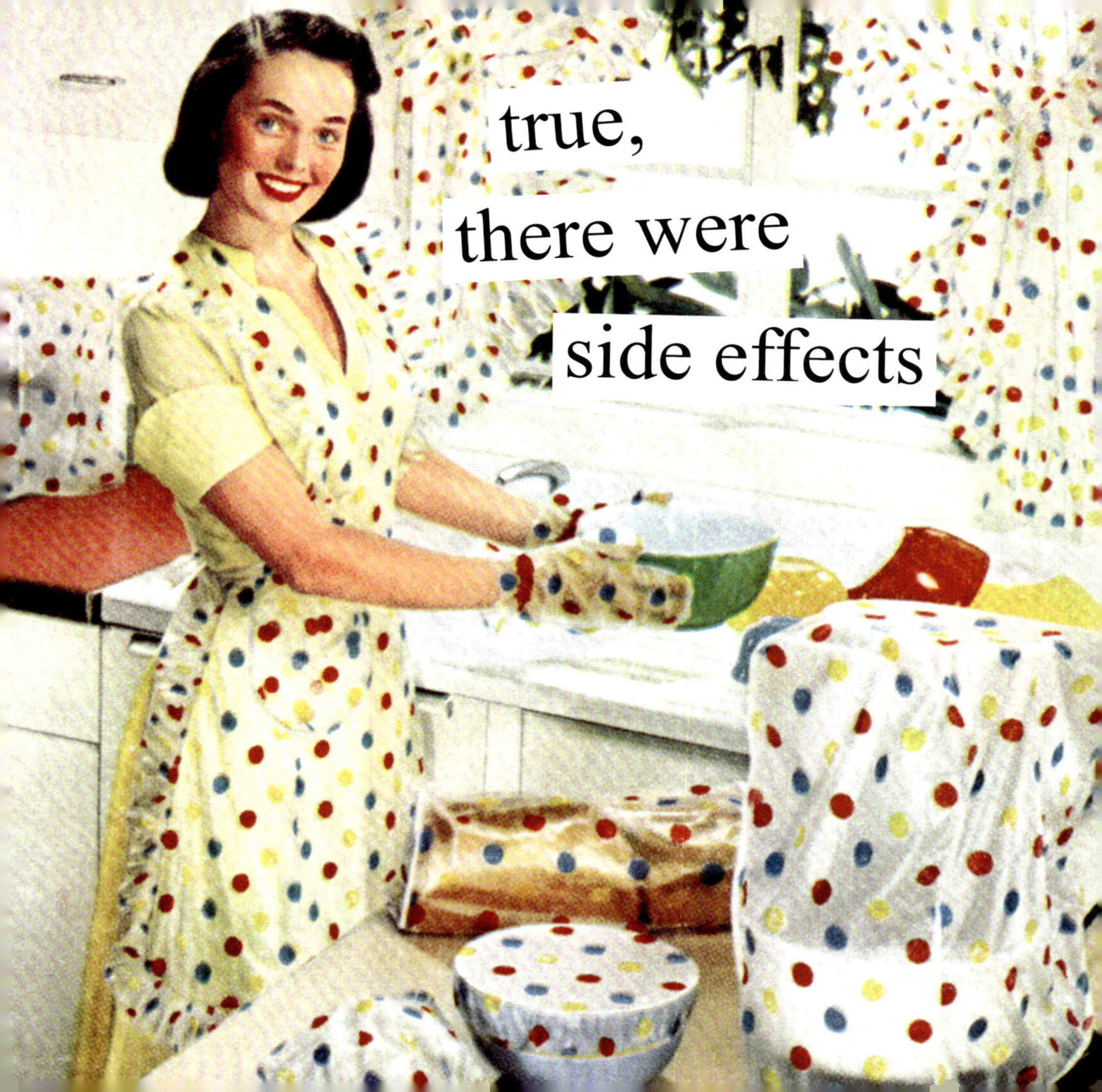
true,
there were
side effects

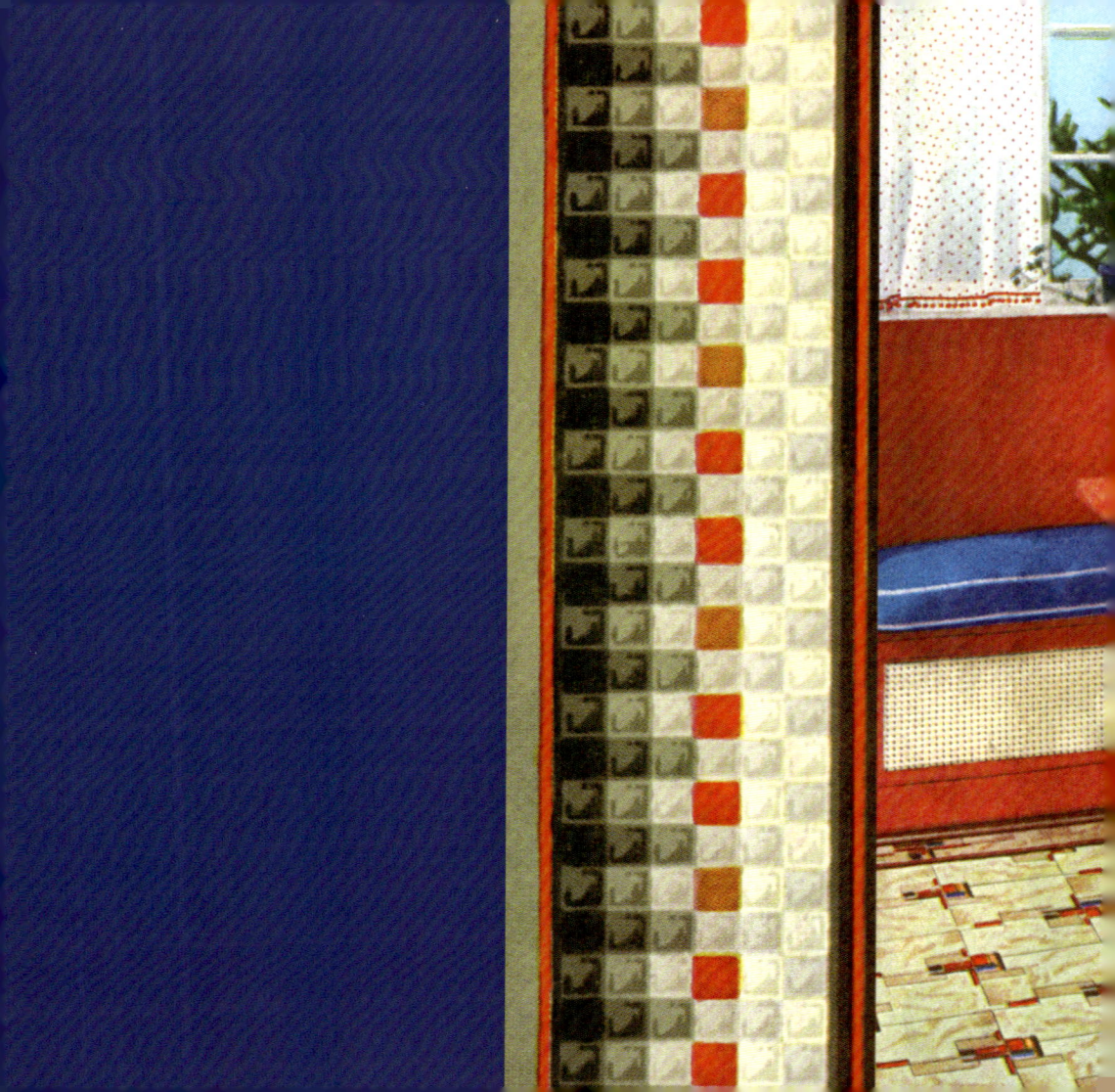

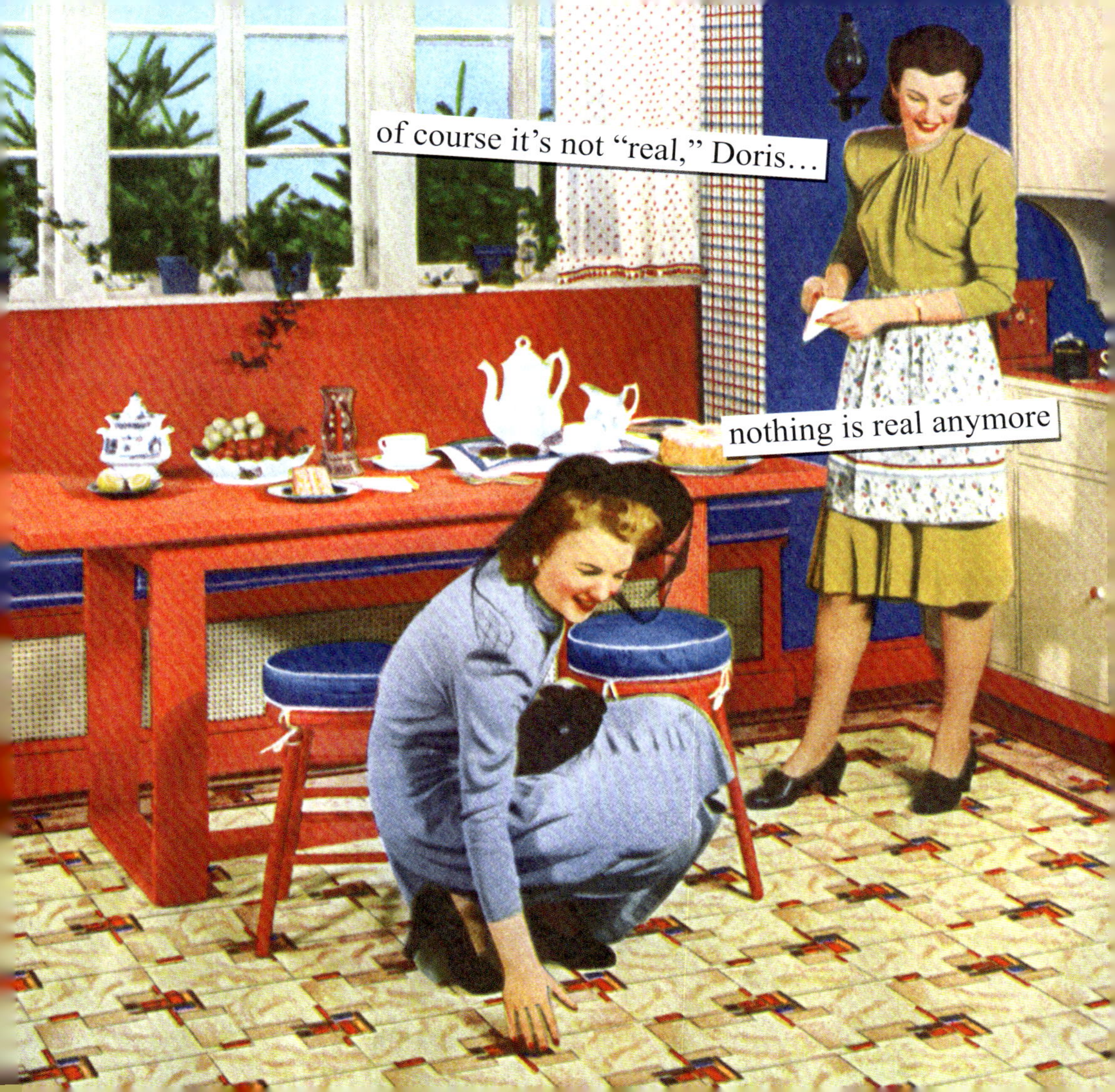
of course it's not "real," Doris…
nothing is real anymore

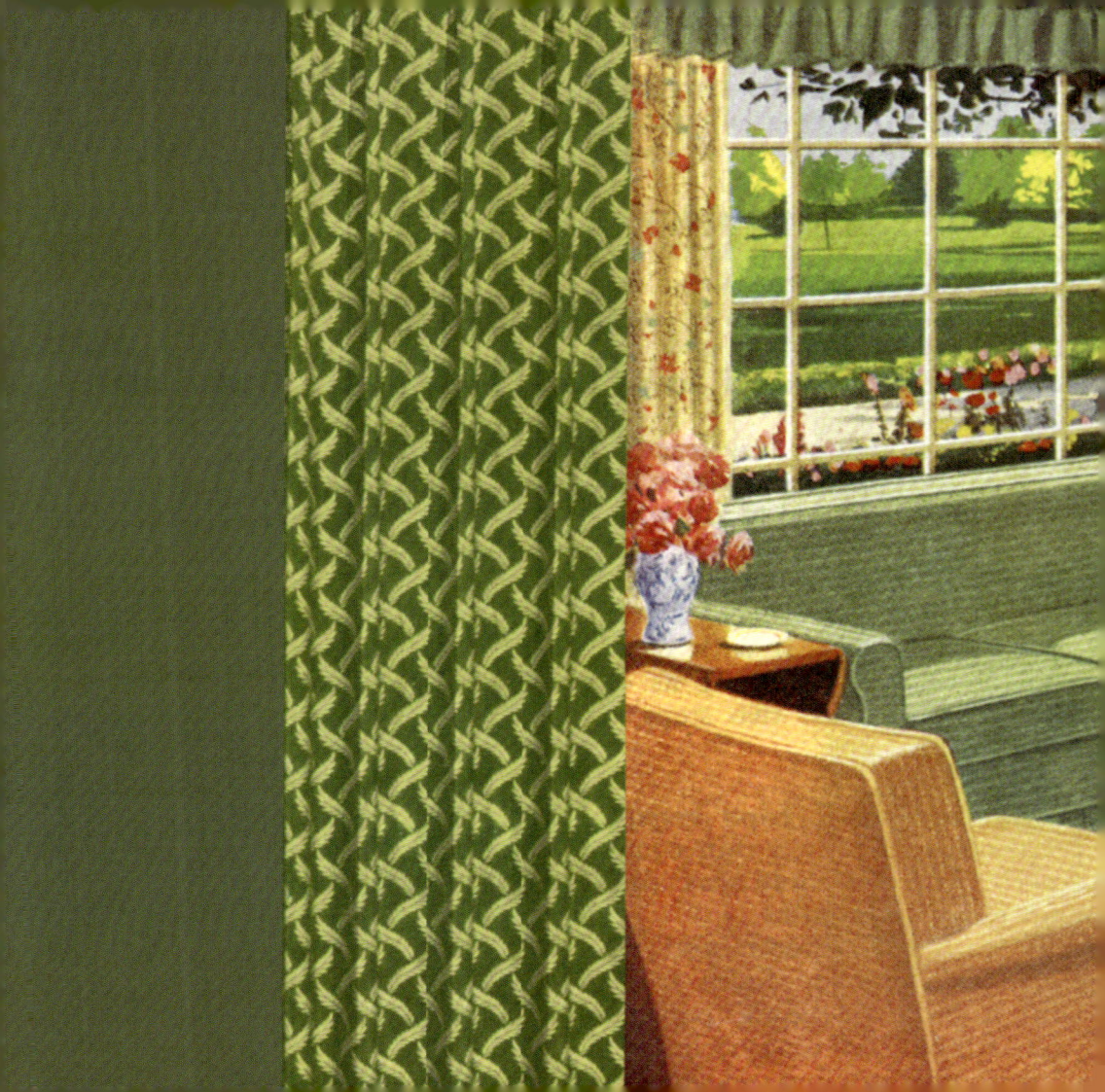

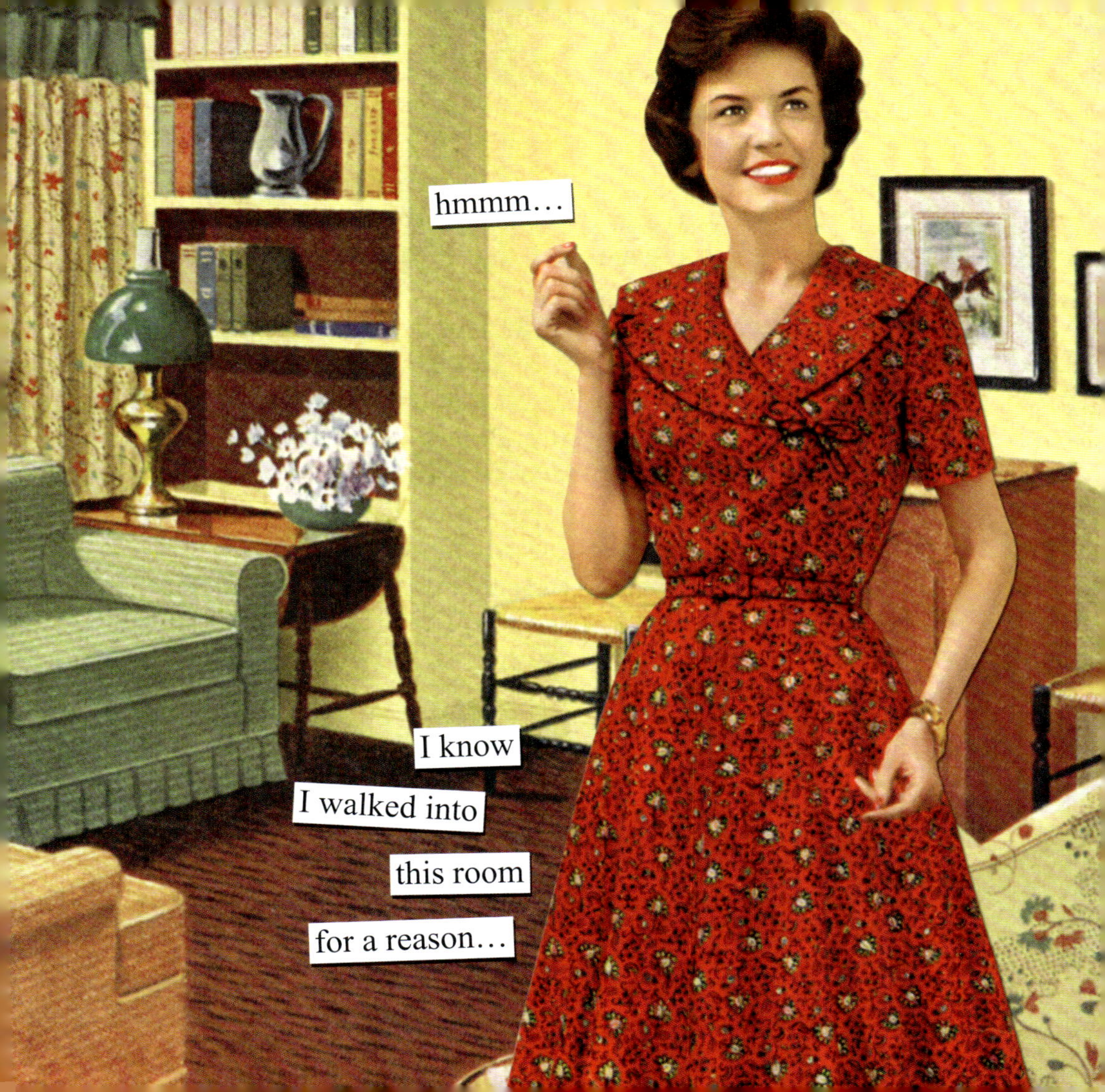
hmmm…
I know
I walked into
this room
for a reason…

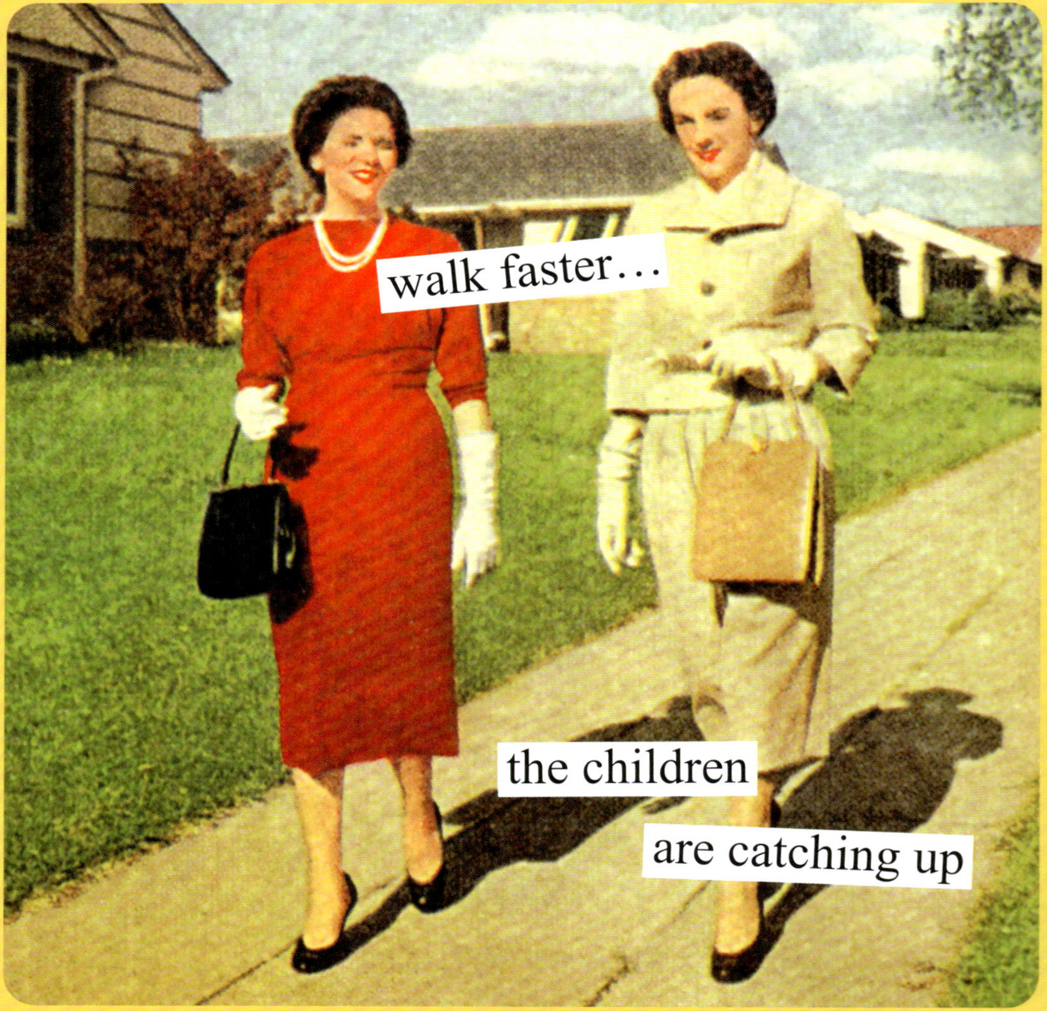
walk faster…
the children
are catching up

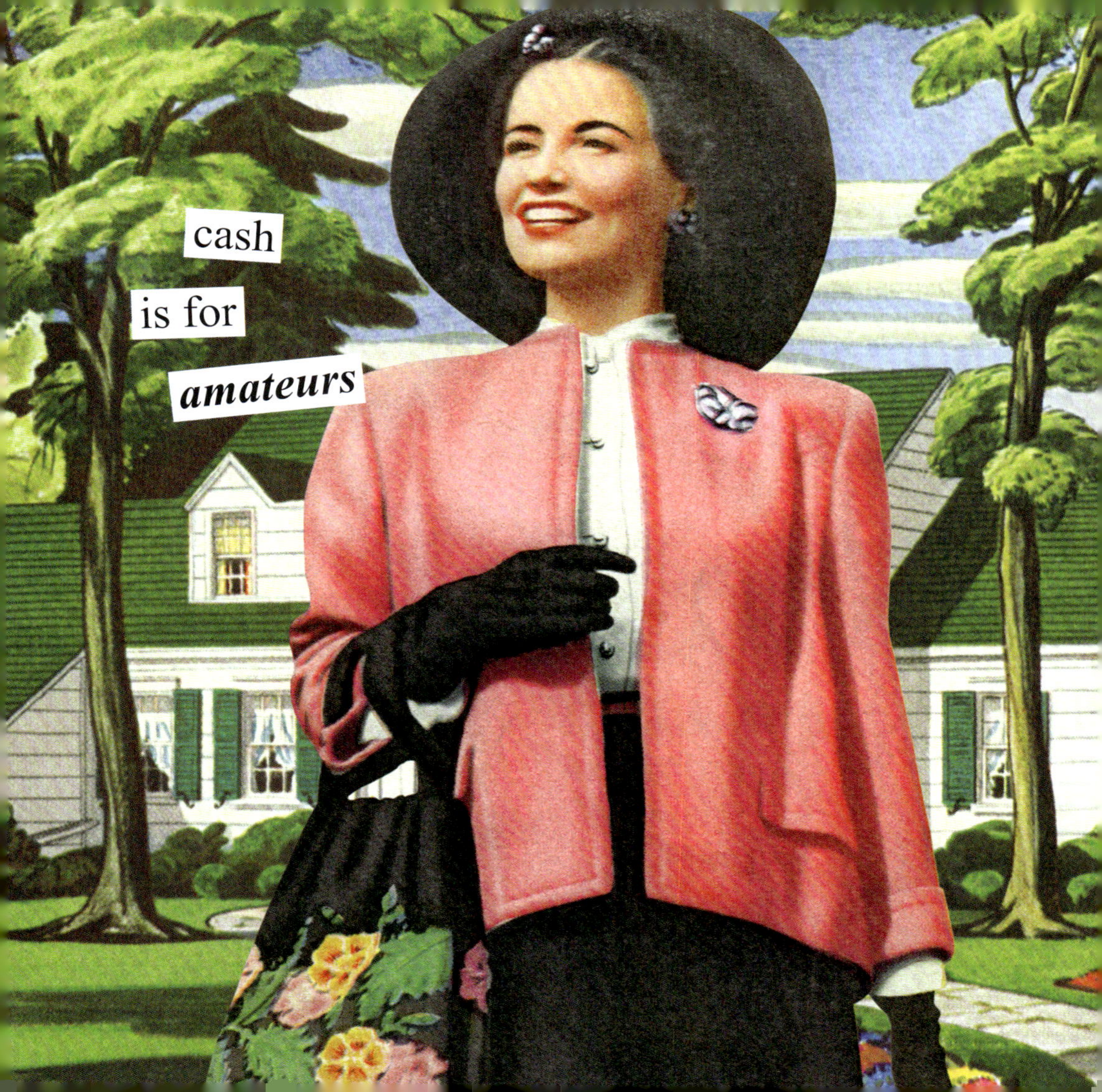

cash
is for
amateurs

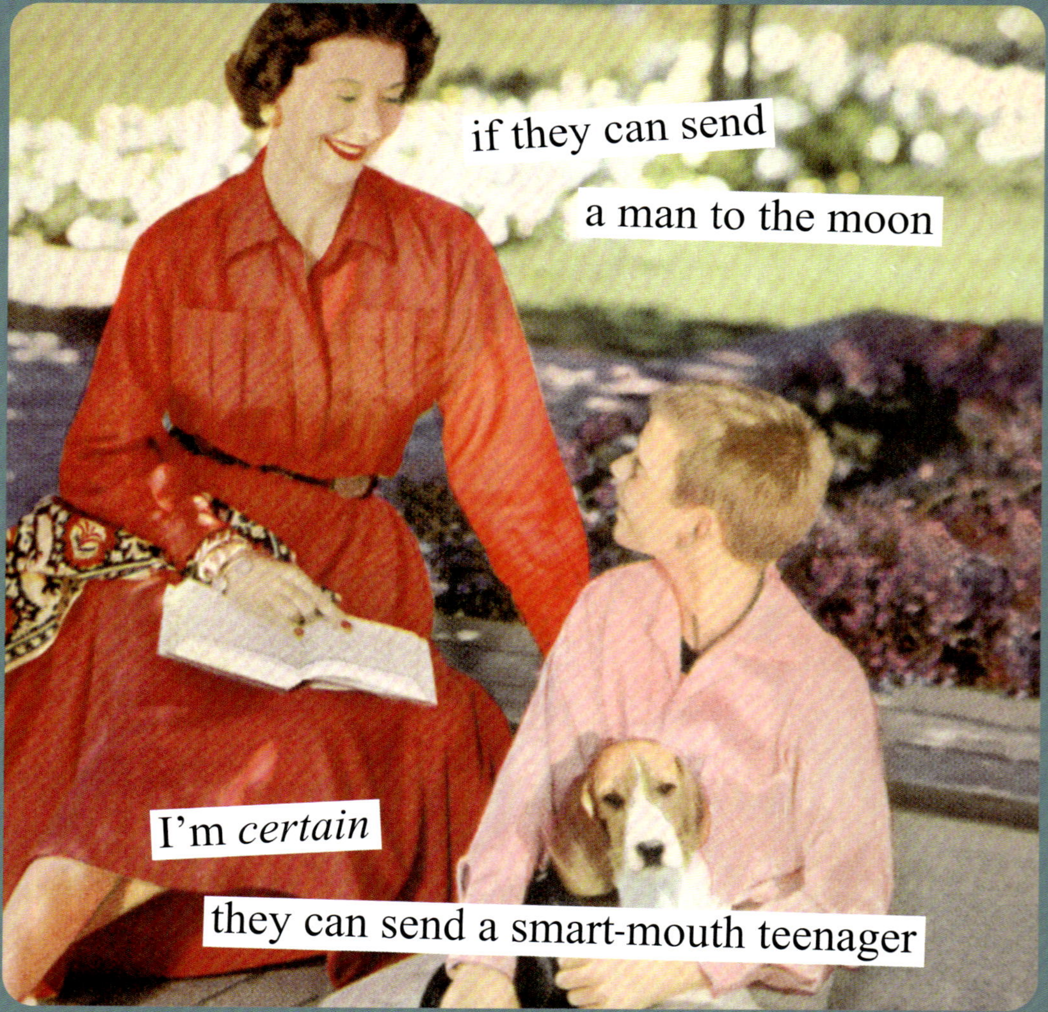
if they can send
a man to the moon
I'm *certain*
they can send a smart-mouth teenager

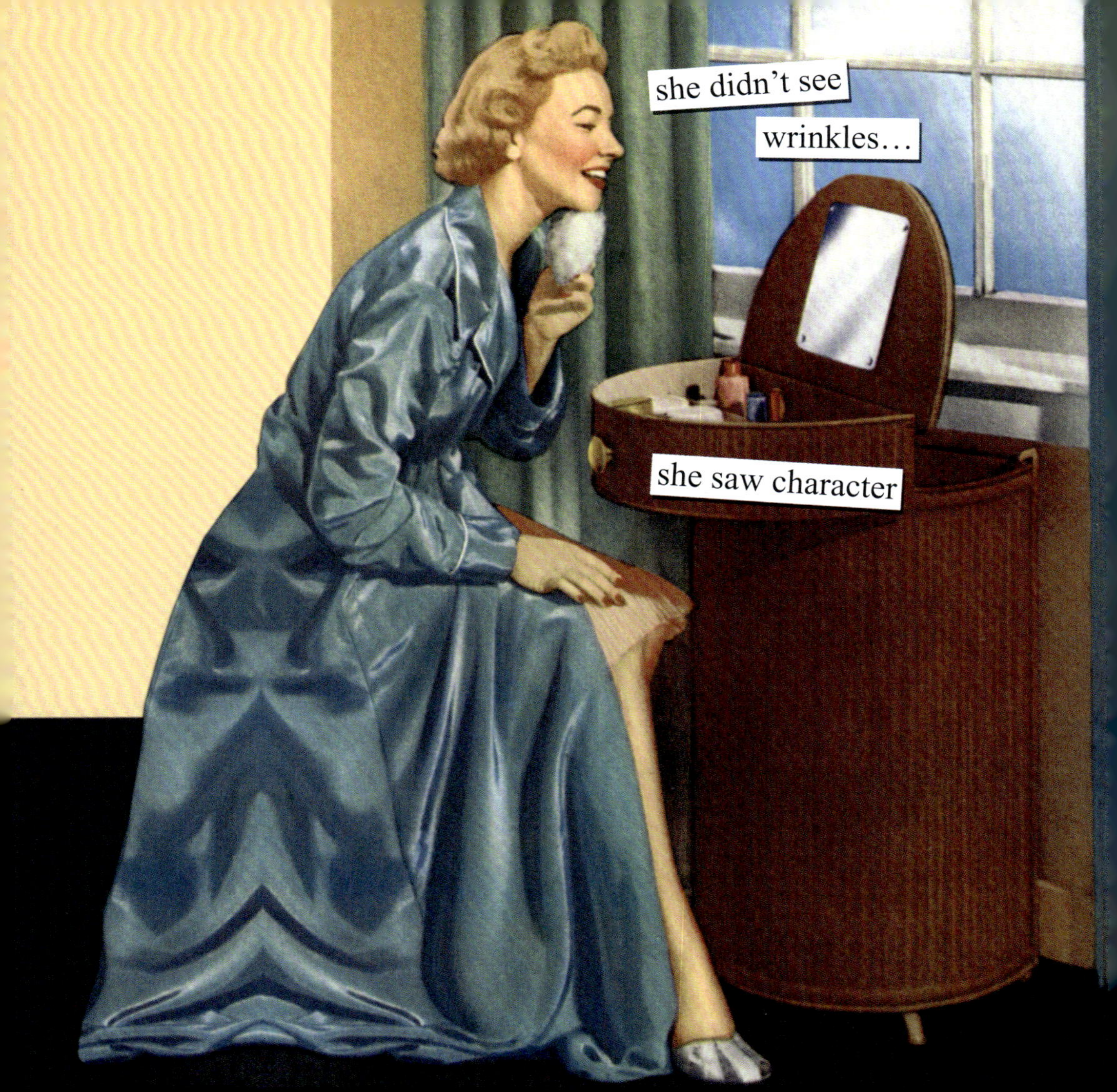
she didn't see
wrinkles…
she saw character

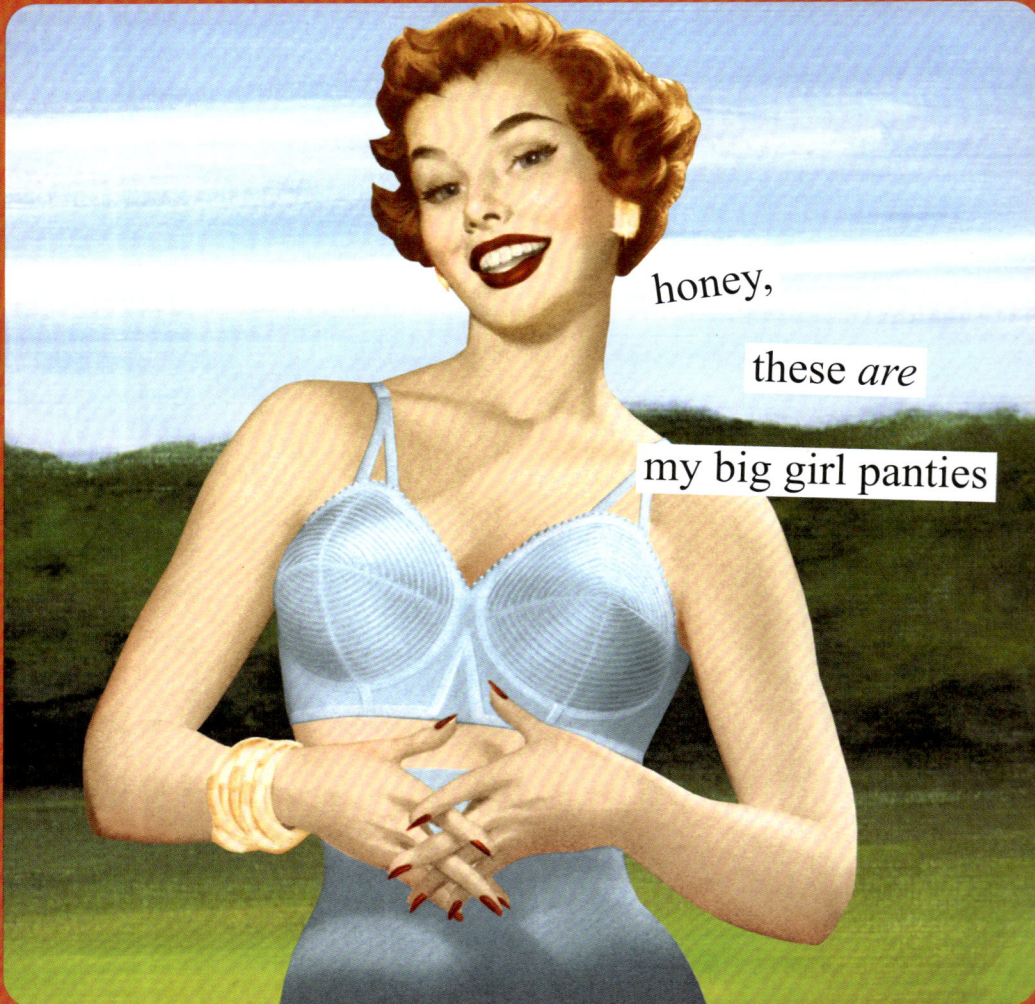

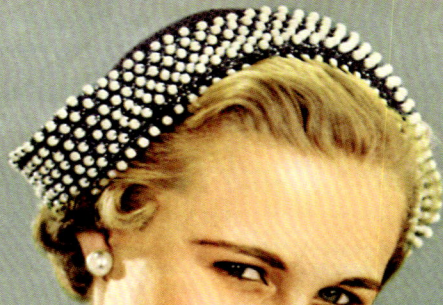

...and best of all

is the matching thong

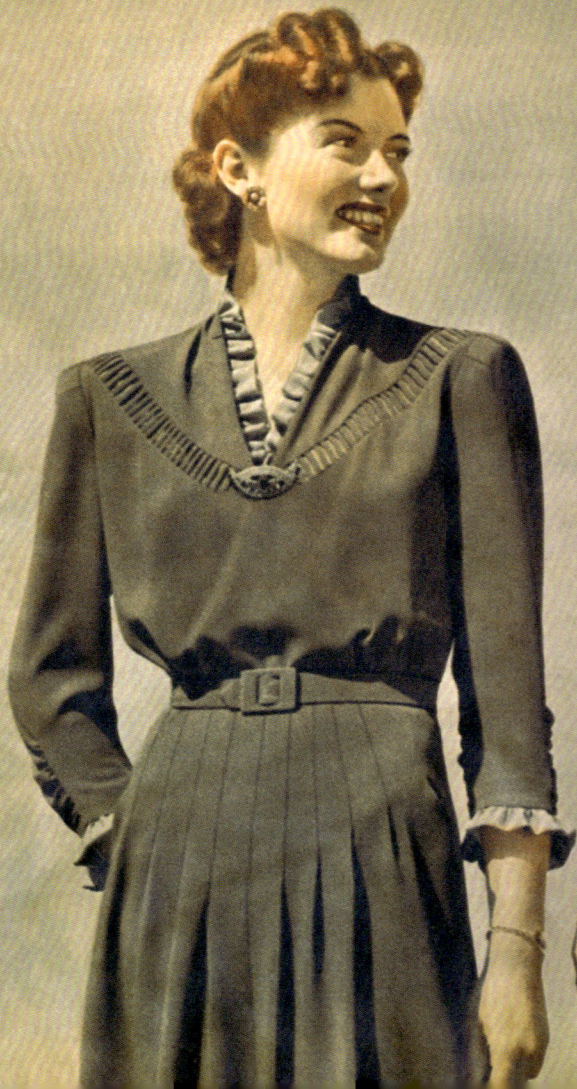

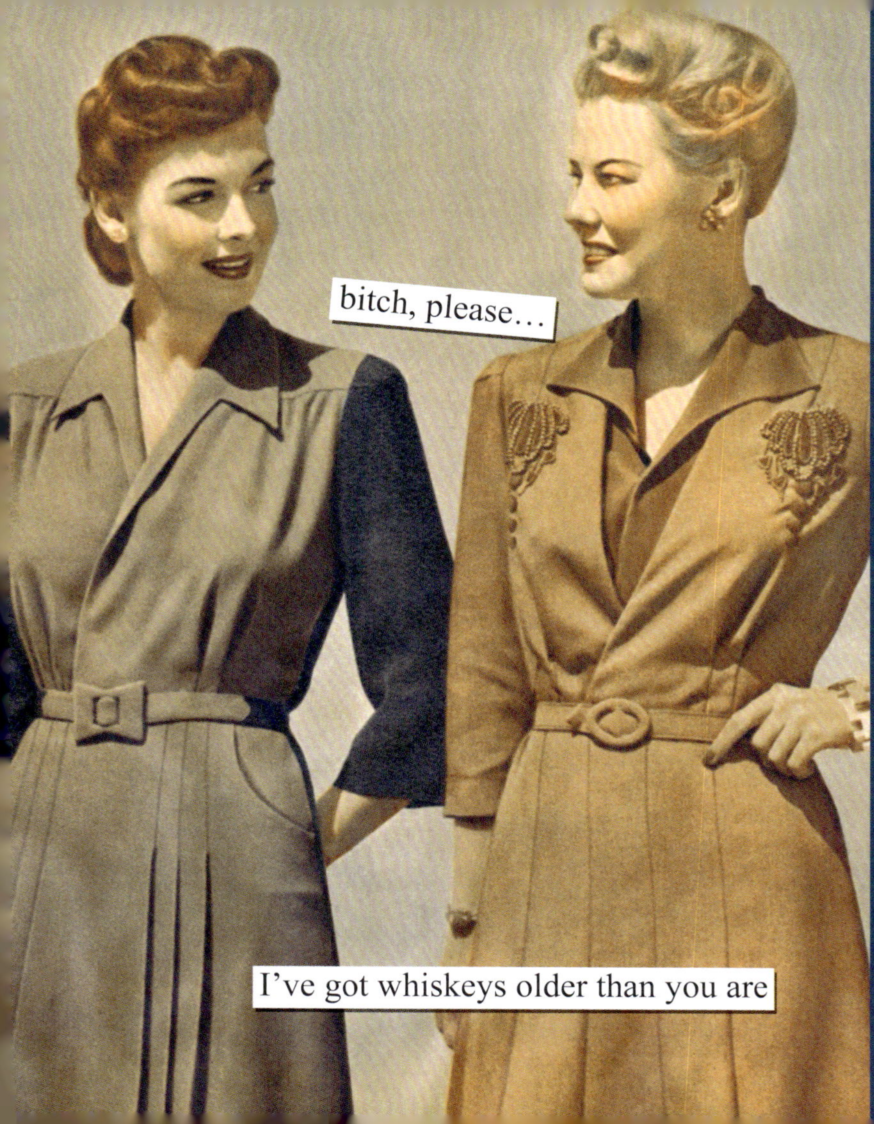
bitch, please…
I’ve got whiskeys older than you are

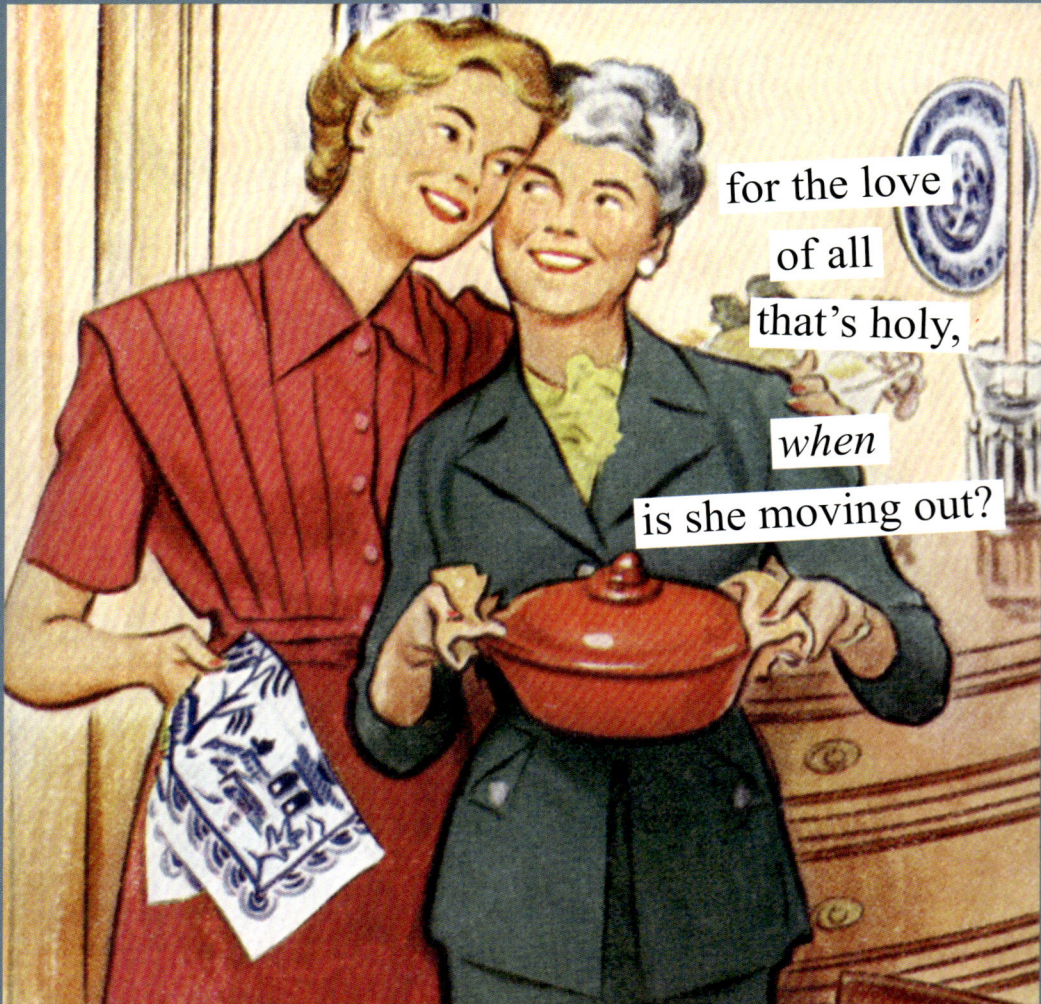

for the love of all that's holy, *when* is she moving out?

God

Bless

This

Empty

Nest

you're never too old…

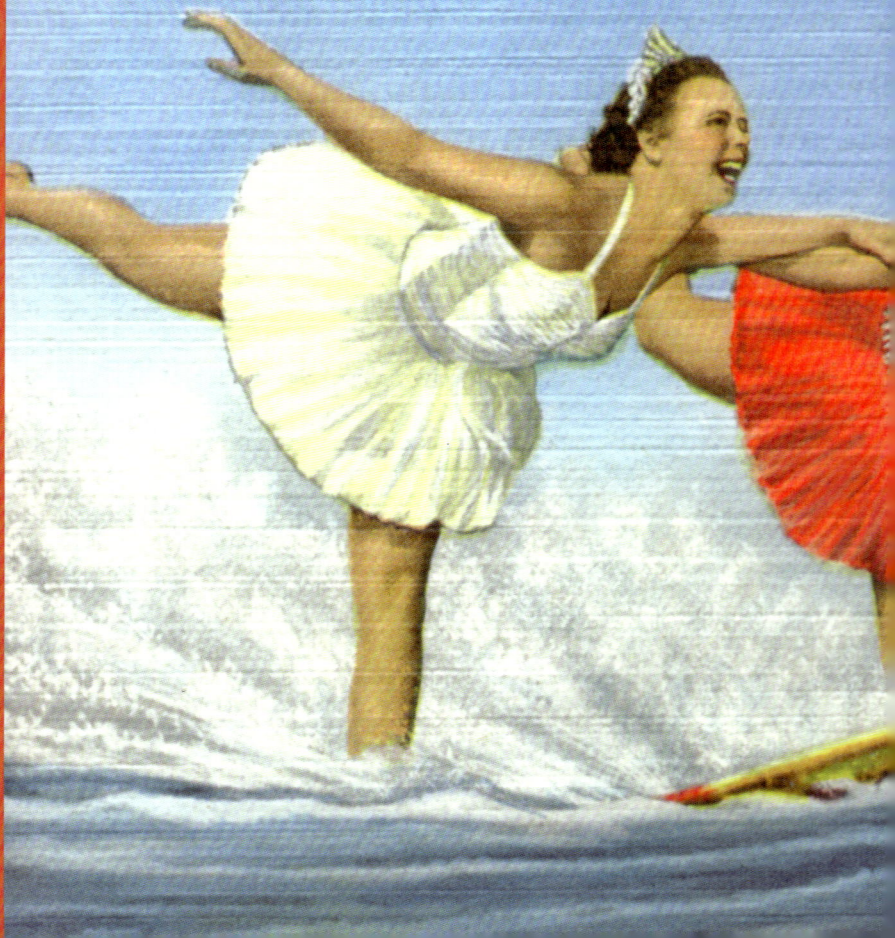

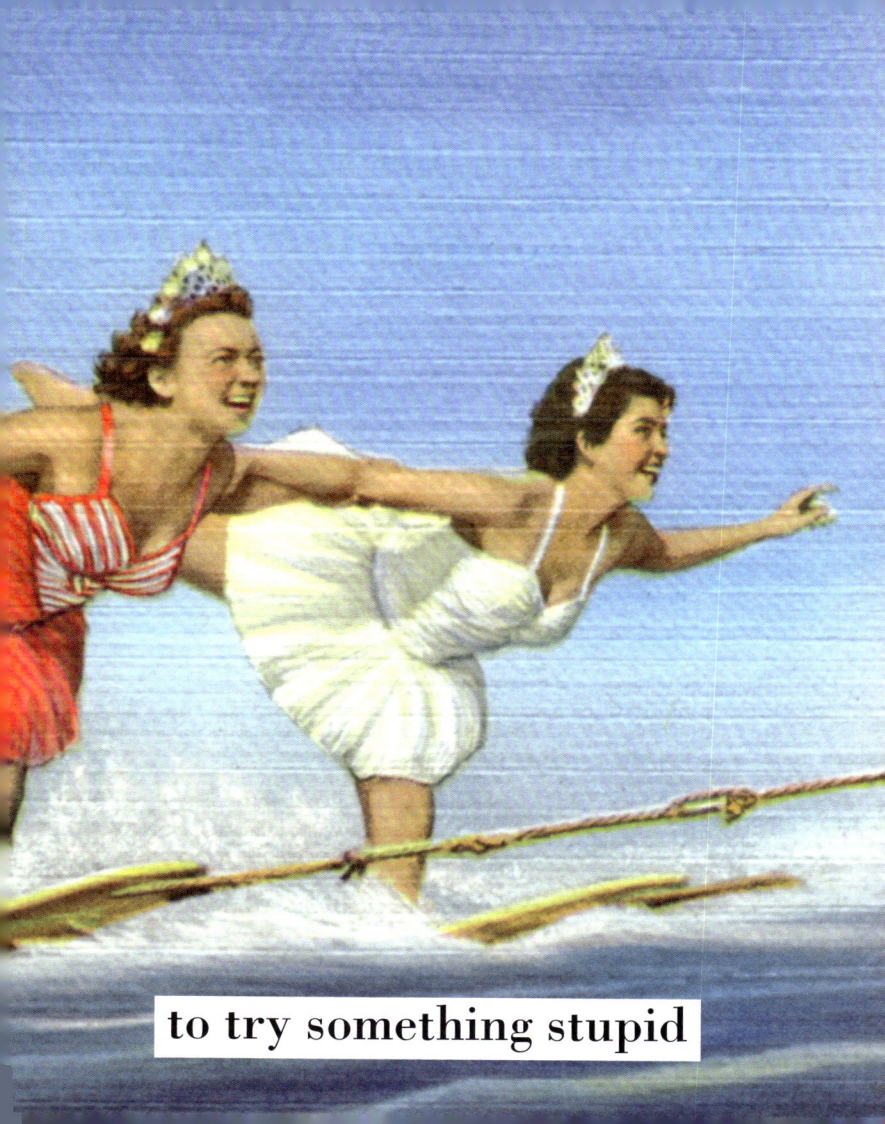

to try something stupid

with age

comes wisdom

big whoop

my garden
kicks
ass

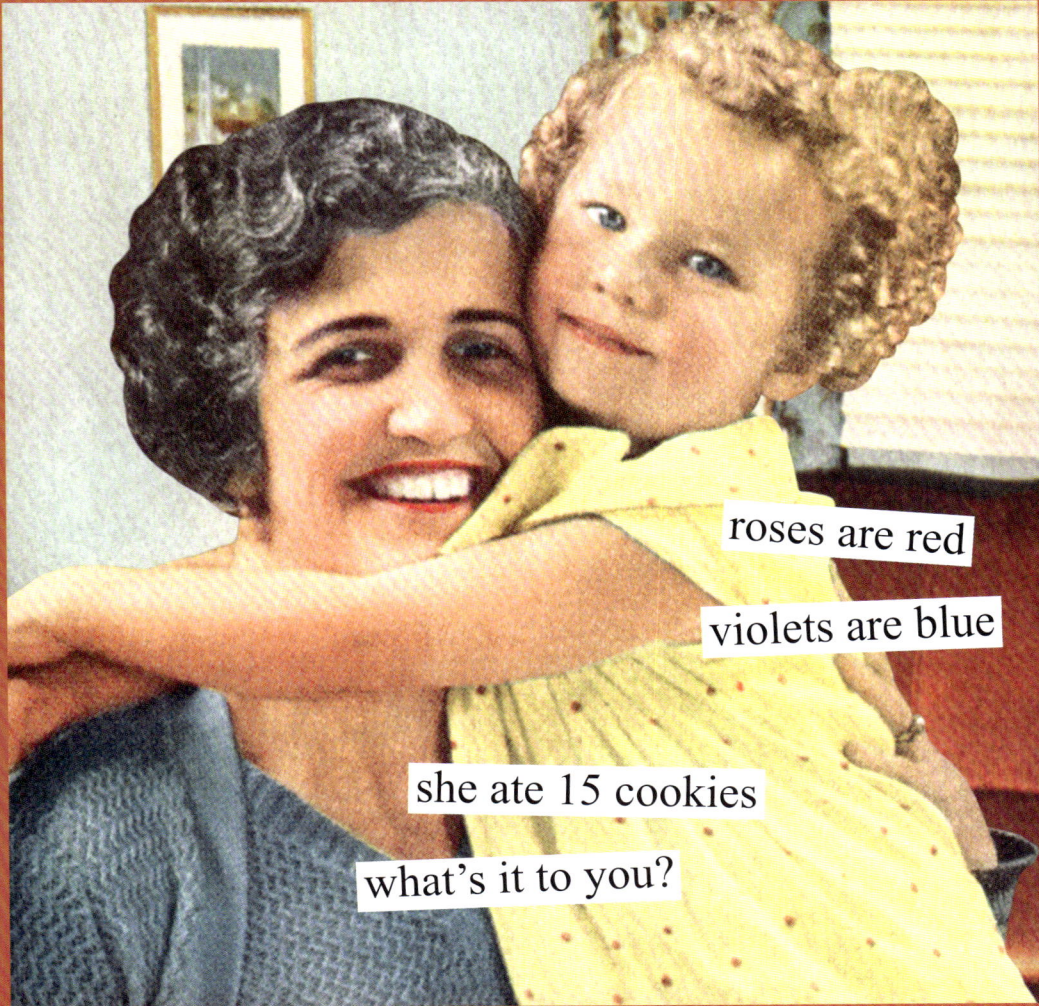

roses are red

violets are blue

she ate 15 cookies

what's it to you?

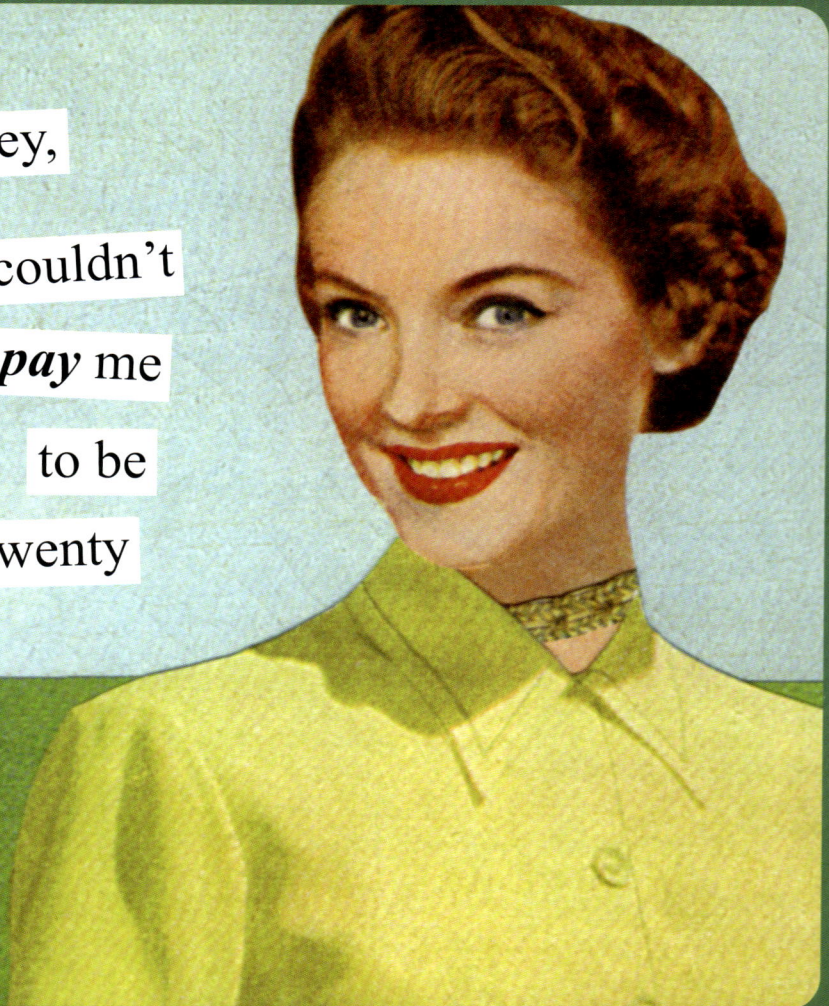

honey,

you couldn't

pay me

to be

twenty

the best thing

about getting old

is forgetting how old you are

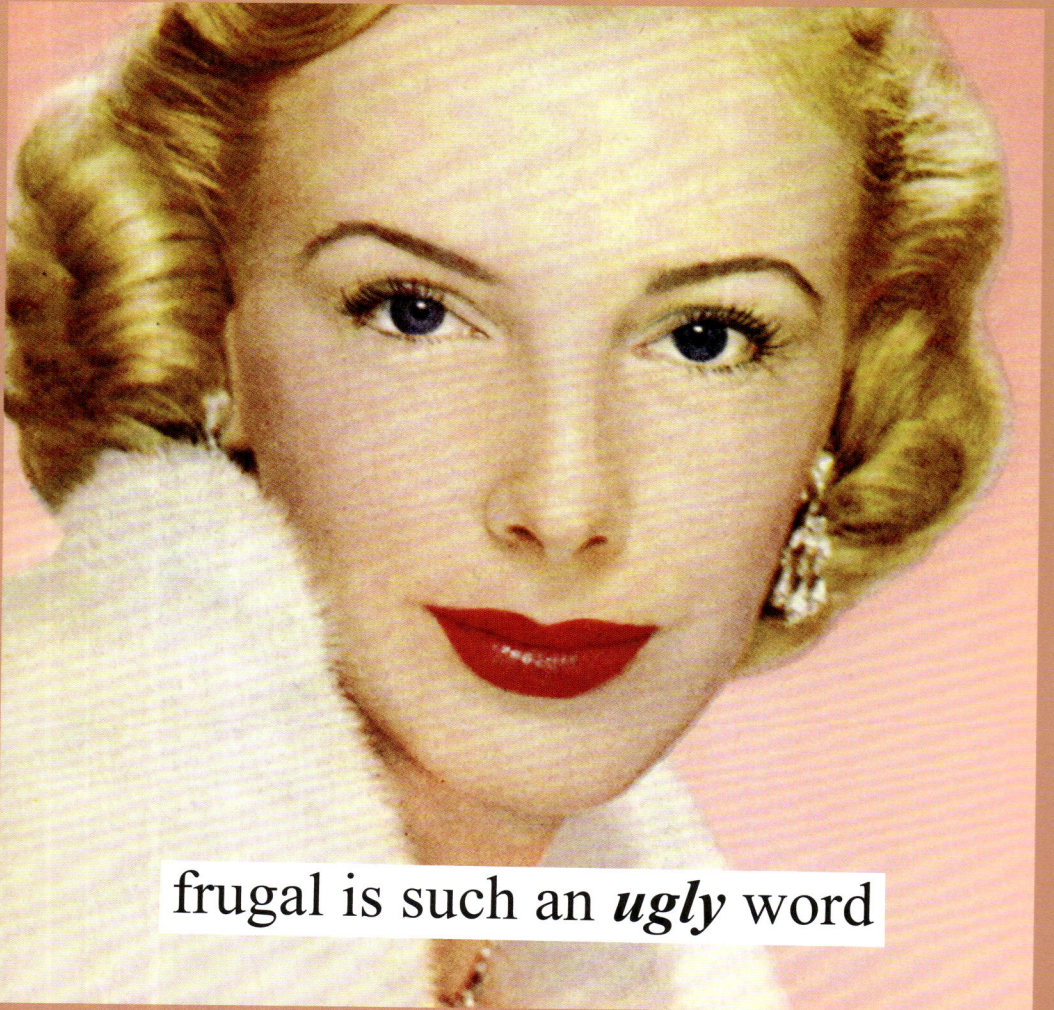

frugal is such an *ugly* word

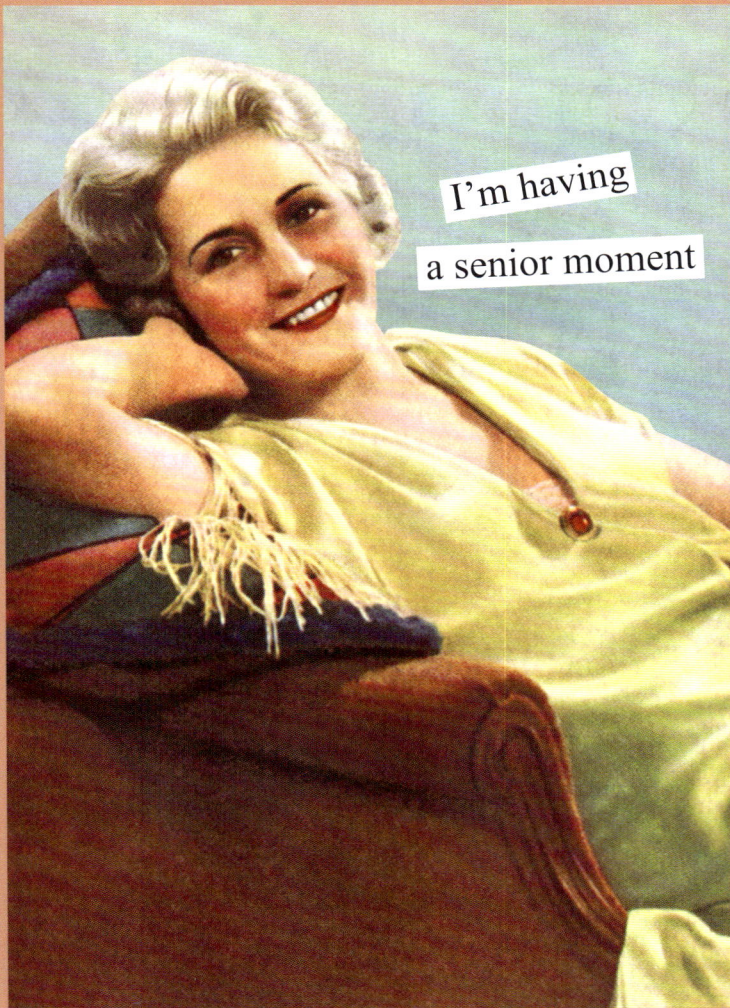

I'm having a senior moment

she could see

no good reason

to act her age

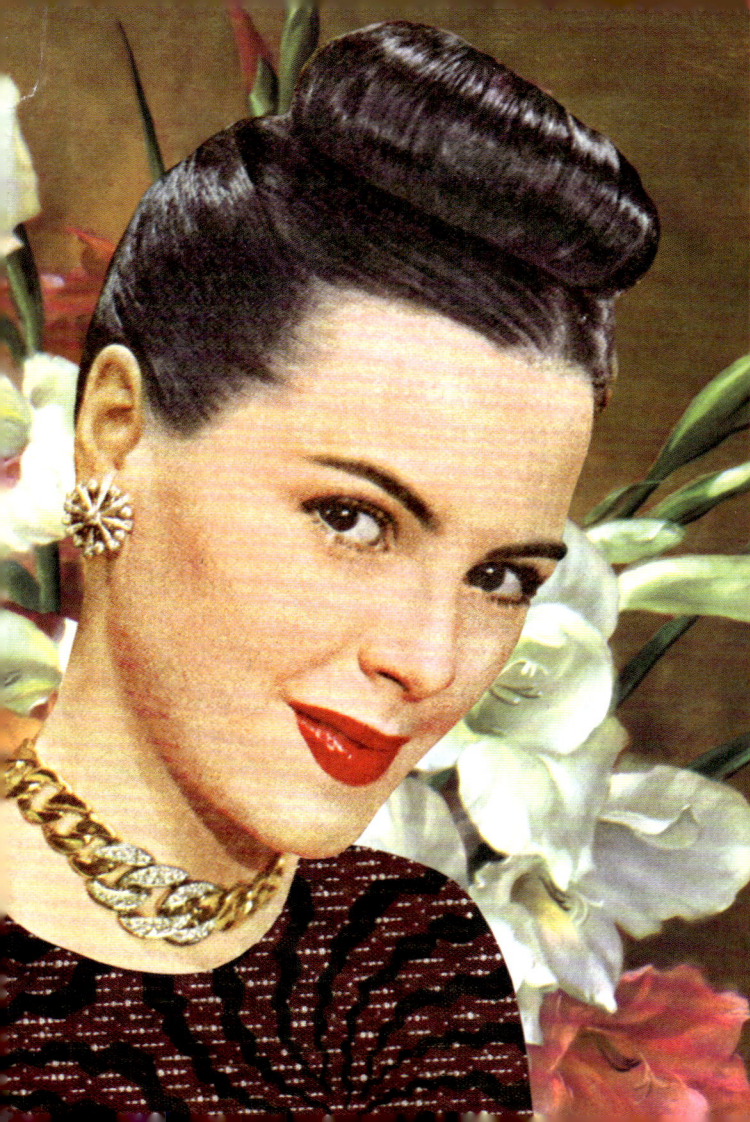

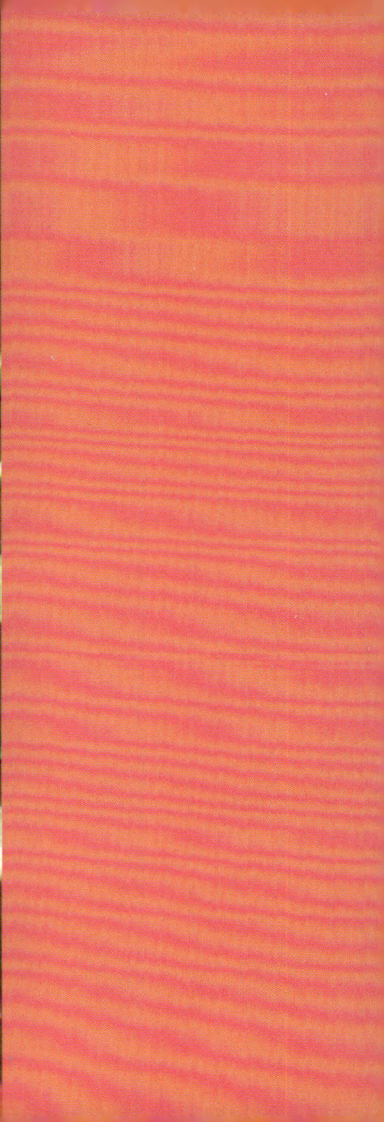

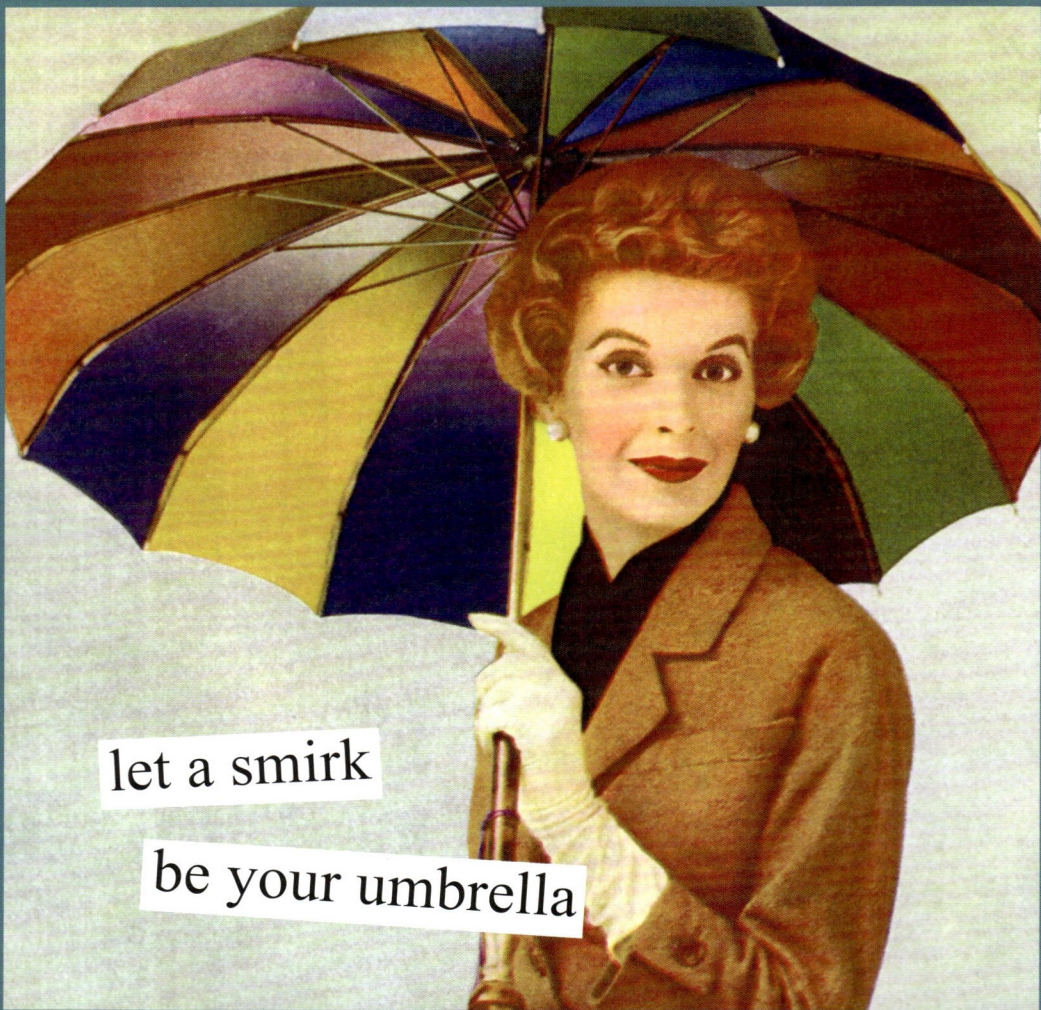

let a smirk

be your umbrella